decluttered

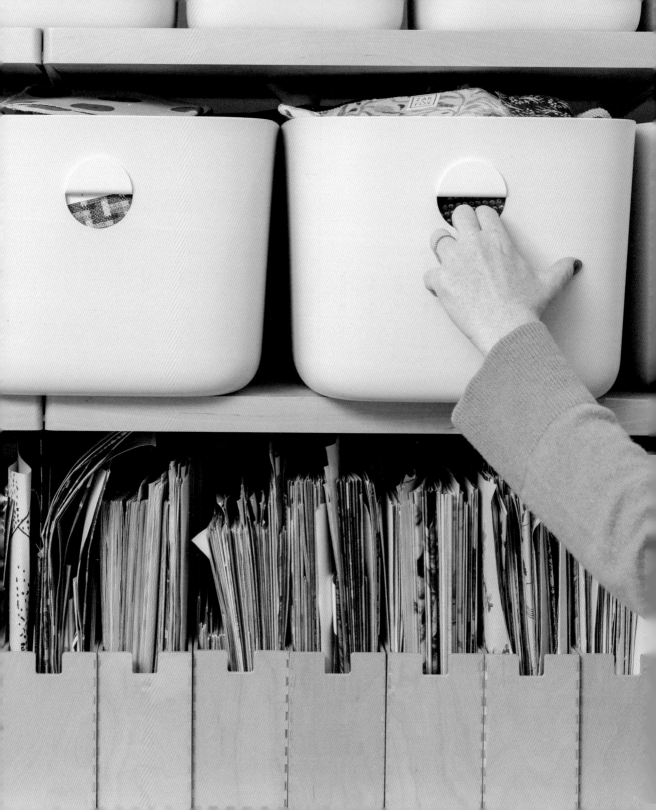

decluttered

Mindful Organizing for Health, Home, and Beyond

JENNY ALBERTINI, MPH

Photography by Birch Thomas

RED LIGHTNING BOOKS

This book is a publication of

Red Lightning Books
1320 East 10th Street
Bloomington, Indiana 47405 USA
redlightningbooks.com

Manufactured in the United States of America

First printing 2024

Cataloging information is available from the Library of Congress.
ISBN 978-1-68435-224-1 (hardback)
ISBN 978-1-68435-226-5 (ebook)

For my clients and
everyone else trying to
get to the bottom of the
clutter in their lives

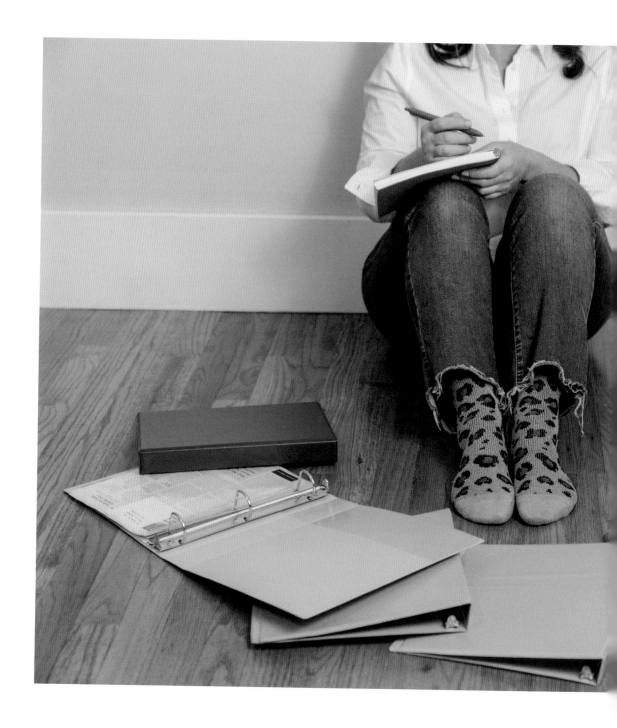

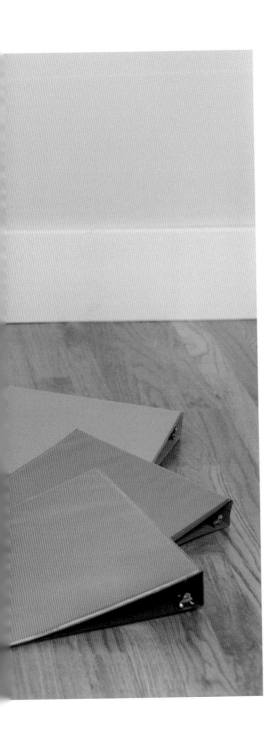

CONTENTS

AUTHOR'S NOTE

Storytelling—both mine and that of people I've worked with—is a central part of this book because our lived experiences best explain how health and clutter intertwine. My clients inspire me, and every day, I see myself in them. Some of their stories are shared here, although I have, of course, changed their names and any identifying details. At times, when common themes emerged, I wove together details from multiple experiences.

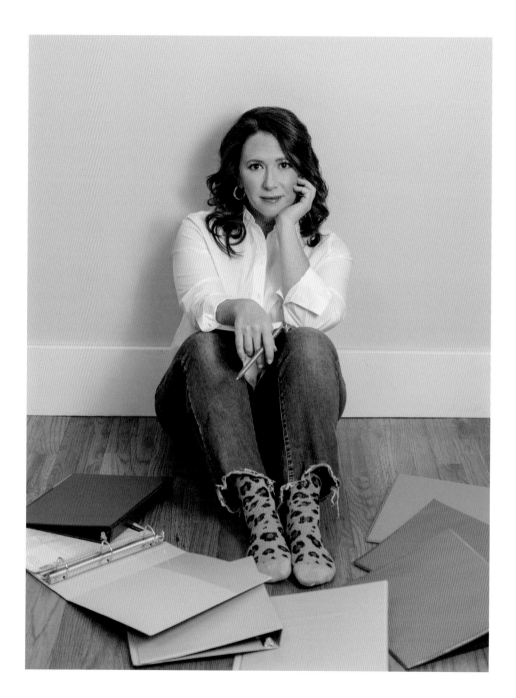

INTRODUCTION

It Starts with a Mess

When I quit a high-level public health job to become a professional home organizer in 2016, I startled people. I had worked at the Centers for Disease Control and Prevention (CDC) and various other government offices and nonprofit organizations for years. Now I was leaving it all behind to train with a Japanese decluttering guru whose main goal was to "spark joy" around the world. I surprised myself, too, as I packed up stacks of research papers and personnel files to clear my desk.

It turned out to be the best decision I'd ever made. Although I didn't recognize it at the time, I needed a radical change. I needed to declutter my life—my whole life. It was not only a career shift for me: it was the start of a years-long process to realign my values with the mental and physical spaces where I spent time. Before making the leap, my well-being was as tumultuous as the places where I spent my time. Earlier in 2016 I had been in a new job where my main duty was to advocate for programs I didn't think were good anymore, and to fill out personnel files on staff members who *definitely* weren't sparking joy anymore. On top of that job, my romantic relationship was sputtering toward a breakup, and close friends of mine started going through a divorce, which ended when one of them died by suicide.

Joy? I didn't know her.

I had read Marie Kondo's *The Life-Changing Magic of Tidying Up* years earlier and loved Kondo's calming presence that came through the pages. She gave people a clear and simple structure to follow to address what was going on in their homes. I'd always loved organizing stuff—first the dollhouse furniture in the yellow, four-room, miniature house I spent hours with after elementary school and, later on, the closets and cupboards in the homes of my friends. Two decades of working on global healthcare initiatives was definitely not bringing me joy anymore, but I was still passionate about health and wanted to help people. While to some the jump seemed like a quantum leap, it made sense to me: I knew clutter was related to health issues, and I wanted to help people transform how that materialized in their lives. But first, I needed to reexamine my own life.

While on vacation in Spain that summer with my soon-to-be-ex boyfriend, I got an email that Kondo was accepting registrations for her new training course. I had floated the idea of quitting to become a professional organizer by my boyfriend a month prior, when I had first heard this course was coming. He was *not* into the idea. Luckily, I trusted my gut and signed up anyway. Over the next few weeks, I resigned from my full-time job and found myself in the basement of a New York City office building learning how to fold a child's snowsuit into thirds.

Was this joy?

Not really. And the first six months of this new path certainly weren't either. In my rush to start this new "joyful" life, I was very strict in following the KonMari guidelines and dissociated this new pursuit from what I had done in my public health jobs. Instead of leaning on my years spent interviewing patients and getting to the root of their health problems, I was asking very specific and surface-level questions about the clutter in clients' homes. I berated myself for not knowing how to attract clients to this new way of organizing, as if I hadn't learned anything about marketing from trying to increase condom use in reproductive health programs for years.

At first, I fought to keep all the parts of me separate—oh, that's Public Health Jenny, this is Organizing Jenny. I had chosen this new thing, so that old thing doesn't matter anymore.

Except I really liked that old thing! Even when I was decluttering my books, I let go of 90 percent of my public health textbooks—no one really needs old biostatistics textbooks—because they didn't bring me joy, but there were some that I kept, usually books telling stories about people and places intersecting around complex human problems and the desire to find a path forward.

More importantly, I reminded myself that I had learned these principles. They were inside me already. I had thought I was a failure because I left my public health career, only to realize that all of that knowledge and experience I had gained and practiced around protecting and improving the health of people and communities was now my superpower for the clients I was working with in their homes and offices. Clutter influences people's health. People's health influences the amount of clutter they have. I began recognizing health problems in the medicine cabinets filled with anxiety pills. I began seeing negotiation scenarios play out in relationships: who was buying the groceries, and who was cleaning the home? I began watching work projects take longer than they should have because no system was in place.

Suddenly it wasn't that I had let Public Health Jenny down; I had found a way to let her out. The more time I spent in people's closets, the more I saw their clutter as a public health problem. The more I analyzed the workplaces I had been in, the more I saw the same combination of issues present. The more I started to bring all of myself to my personal and professional interactions, the closer I got to people—and the closer I got to the problems plaguing so many of us.

Then in 2020, the pandemic charged the intensity of what was going over everyone's doorstep. Stepping over the thresholds every day into my clients' homes was already complicated and now, health issues and inequities were exacerbated. As these problems became magnified by the global media, there was increasing awareness of how integrated issues of health, home and structural choices and circumstances were—thus affecting the wherewithal of my clients to live comfortable lives every day. People were more overwhelmed and unsure than ever about where their personal agency began and societal constructs end. They lived among this chaos at home, at work, and in their communities, not unlike how we watched policies, and their consequences play out all around the world at the onset and during the spread of COVID-19. The pandemic reinforced my belief about how uncertainty and disorder can manifest as chaos all around us, suppressing our potential, happiness, and freedom. Almost always, when it comes to decluttering the problem isn't the clutter; the problems are the habits, con-

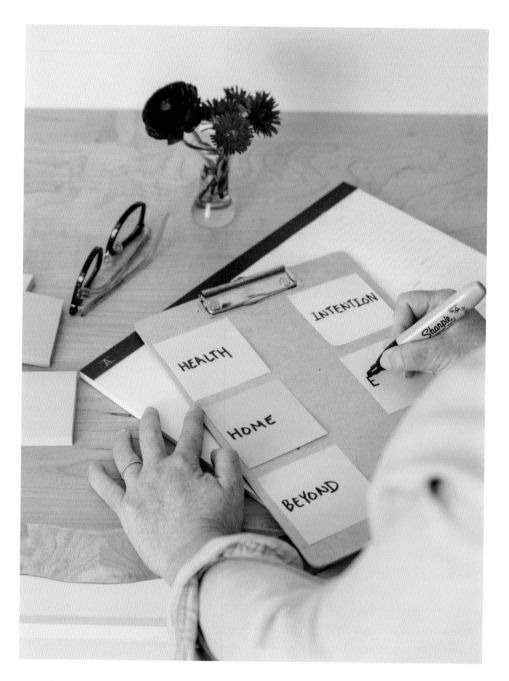

straints, and circumstances of our lives that create the clutter. When we solve those underlying issues, the real change can happen.

When we take the time to explore our relationships to clutter, the possibilities for relief, ease, and joy appear where we least expect them. What brings me joy now? Many things, but one of the best sources, one that always makes me smile, is when I hear from clients who *finally* feel organized in their homes or family lives because they were able to prioritize their health. Or the reverse: a client who feels great about their health because they *finally* live in an environment that meets their needs.

I'm glad I left that government job a few years back, and it's OK that it took me a little while to figure out how to feel like myself in my new role. It makes my confidence so much stronger now. I am still decluttering my life in little ways here and there, reassessing my needs and wants. It's an ongoing journey, and I'm here to help you start yours.

This book is a guide for people who are on a journey of mindfully organizing their lives. It recognizes the complexity of the different circumstances for readers and is written with compassion—and occasional humor—in mind. Decluttering is about so much more than getting rid of things. When we make purposeful choices about what we want to live with, we also set intentions for how we want to live. When we make purposeful choices about our relationships to the home, we also set intentions for what the home feels like. When we make purposeful choices about who we want to work with, we also set intentions for how we want to work. This book is for people who are ready to transform their relationships, their homes, their workplaces, and their societies one "next best step" at a time.

My goal is to provide context around why different types of clutter affect all areas of our lives—our health, our homes, and our personal and professional goals, the latter of which I will refer to as "the beyond" throughout the book. I believe we can take steps to alleviate the harm clutter causes by using a public health approach, which involves defining and measuring the problem, determining the cause or risk factors for the problem, figuring out how to prevent or mitigate the problem, implementing effective strategies on a larger scale, and evaluating the impacts of those strategies. Don't worry though, no PhD needed here; I've taken these scientific concepts and crafted them into easy-to-follow exercises. Whether you have the urge to address something right in front of you, like your kitchen, or something more abstract, like the benefits program at your workplace, it's vital to understand how they are all related and what steps you can take to work on them based on your energy and agency for any given situation.

Making a kitchen or spare bedroom look nice is fine, but I'm most interested in why decluttering makes people feel better—and what they can do with that improved sense of self. Mindful and personal, my process is grounded in the KonMari Method™ of tidying up and informed by a deep understanding of how the environment impacts our health and well-being. While the result of our work can be seen all around you, my approach addresses the unseen root causes of excess. In that way, there is no other book quite like the one you have found yourself reading now.

Working with community-health leaders, politicians, and hospital administrators, I learned to create behavioral-change programs for health and wellness settings around the world. In each case, we prioritized the patient experience, ensuring the programs were designed to meet patient needs and aligned with scientifically proven best practices. I bring the same compassionate and analytical approach to my work with my clients—using proven methods to achieve lasting results and setting goals that are both manageable and sustainable.

When we only change our environments, we aren't changing our habits, yet habits are where life-altering transformation begins, as I've seen proven out in the field—in this case, the home and the office. The mindful decluttering and organizing strategies we'll practice together in this book try to make these behavioral changes as creative, painless, and transformative as possible.

My process asks you to peel back the layers of clutter in your life to understand where it's stemming from in the first place. The experience is emotional, physical, and enlightening. Over time, and with dedication, we can reveal what's going on beneath the surface and provide an opportunity for you to change your circumstances for the better—and for good. As we transform what's going on inside of us, our physical spaces shift around us too . . . once and for all.

That's why it's so important to not just sweep through your space and race to clean up or throw out what bothers you in the moment. Instead, I'll be asking you to go slower and look deeper, to uncover how you've created the life around you and what changes you want to

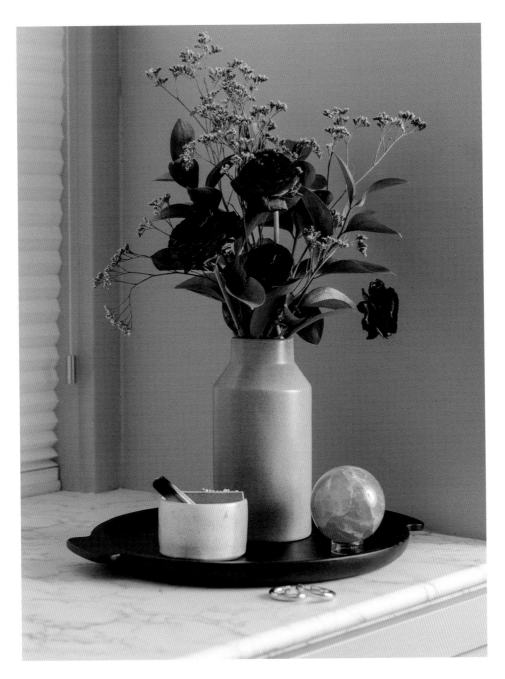

experience. When you do, you'll see what you've really been holding on to—and been held back by.

When you put the time into completing this process, you'll receive time back in return. How? Because you'll minimize roadblocks and simplify processes in your daily life that used to create stress—more stress than this process ever will. You'll also create new mindful habits that support and sustain the change you've established.

Decluttered is not:

- a guide on shelf styling,
- a list of the best wellness supplements, or
- a trick to get your boss to let you work less.

All those things sound wonderful, but good sources for those ideas already exist.

Rather, this book will weave together a new narrative on decluttering, one that is reflexive, proactive, and can be tailored to your unique circumstances.

Decluttered is:

- an examination of how the physical and emotional environments in which we spend our time affect our well-being,
- a menu of options to experiment with to create changes geared toward improving well-being, and
- a system grounded in the knowledge of what constrains us and how we can dismantle those boundaries.

In these pages, you will find stories of clients who experienced tremendous relief after making key changes in their personal, home, and work lives. I've also gone through these stages of change and share my journey too within these pages. You will also find suggestions on how to make educated assessments of what's going on in your life by paying attention in ways that could be different from how you typically do so.

When most people think of decluttering, they focus on the stuff—and the putting away of that stuff. We'll talk about that a bit, of course, but mostly I want us to think more broadly about clutter and try out different ways to get a handle on it so that more areas of your life feel better. To do that, I'm including a series of exercises in each chapter ("Health," "Home," and "Beyond"), which will offer different ways to either learn more about ourselves and how clutter is showing up in our lives or try out specific ways of mitigating the effect clutter is having, through communication strategies, creative activities, and more. These are options for ways to take action, especially with exercises that use different creative modalities and communication scripts to reduce anxiety before tough conversations. I also provide writing exercises with prompts so you can move forward with clarity and intention. Some of these exercises might not seem like what you want to normally do while reading a book—and that's fine. I can't tell whether you do them or not! But I do believe that if you want to feel differently, then you have to try some new ways of being, and one of these "weird" self-experiments might be just the trick to spark that type of idea—if you are committed to clearing the clutter from your life.

When we feel overwhelmed, knowing where to start can be hard. I want you to feel supported at each step with this book. It was written to be read as a whole, but the individual chapters can be useful on their own. If you are focused on addressing feelings of being overwhelmed in any of the three specific areas addressed here (health, home, and beyond), you can turn to those chapters first or individually. Don't forget, though, that if you've been neglecting one of these sections, say your health, and only focusing on clutter you can see in your home, you are likely missing out on the opportunity to address issues that are interrelated. Paying attention to the clutter in all areas of our lives can help balance out how we feel, what we do, and who we are.

Many of us like "real life" examples and templates for how to make changes or have tough conversations, so you'll also see some of those. The personal and client stories I've shared here may feel familiar to you and things you've gone through; I hope these help you feel less alone in your struggle to mindfully organize your life. The mindfulness of this process really takes over when you become present in thinking through and acting on the underlying issues most relevant to your life.

We all deserve to live and work in beautiful, functional spaces. Orderly environments create calm and happiness and allow us to be purposeful in our intentions and actions. It's not just the space around us though that cultivates those feelings though; its also our relationships to the people we spend time with, and to our identity and self-expression in those spaces. We've got a lot of mindful organizing to do to get decluttered . . . so let's get started.

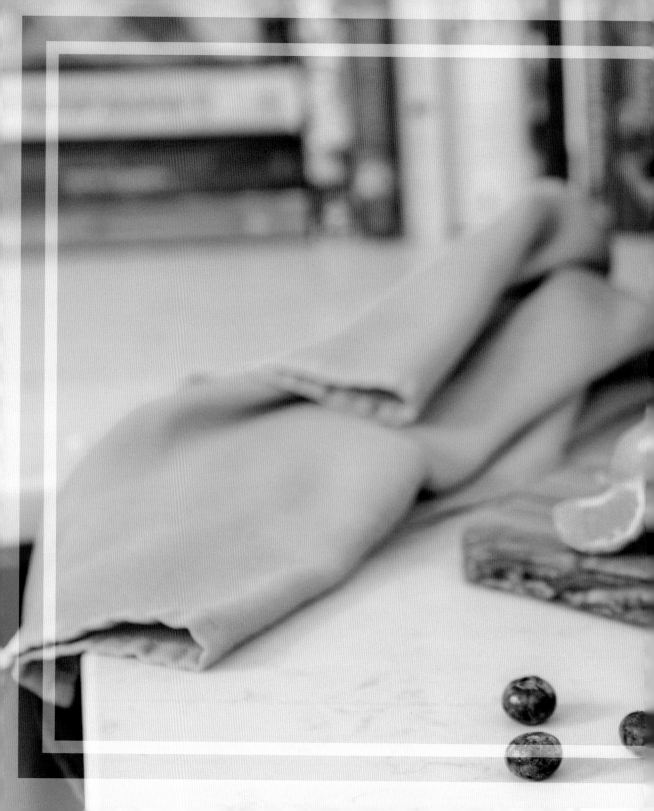

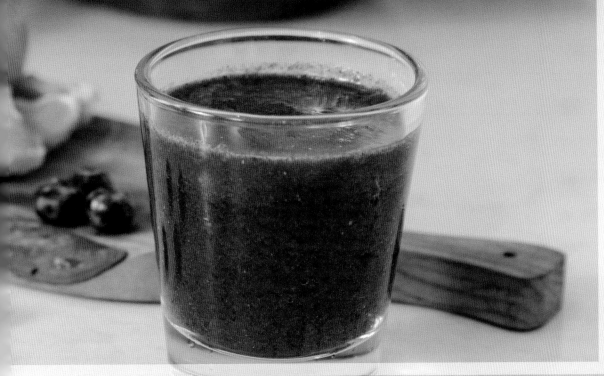

HEALTH

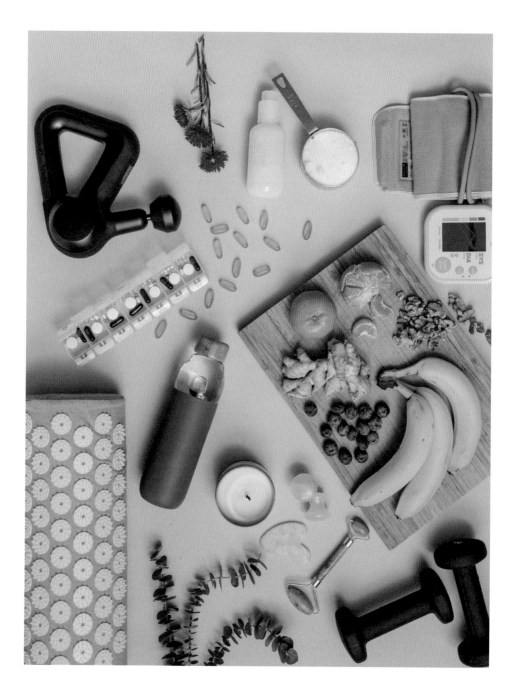

HEALTH

Sara's breathing was rapid, almost keeping pace with her wringing hands. Her eyes darted around the room, avoiding lingering too long on any one spot against the walls, where the problems were piling up. Literally a dozen or so tubs of paper were stacked floor to ceiling against the wall. These tubs she had lugged from apartment to apartment, year after year, were no longer just extra objects to carry up and down stairs. The thousands of notes, bills, and printed-out emails inside them stacked up and over the edges like waves of guilt hurling themselves at her.

Why now? I asked myself. *Why me?* I thought.

Sara had invited me in to hold her hand and guide her, to nudge her from behind and pull her gently ahead on the path of "decisions already made." I was a stranger, save just one phone call before our meeting, with only a website and soothing phone voice to convince her that I could help her solve years' worth of concerns. Walking through her apartment, her brow was furrowed, while I made sure to stay relaxed and open, positive enough for the both of us. I breathed calmly until she could match my rhythm. This last move to DC had brought her enough chutzpah, hope, and promise that she wanted to seize that energy and address whatever the extra-large containers taking up her floor space and stacked high within her closets contained. She wanted to be rid of the anxiety attacks that popped up each time she thought about what might be lurking within the tubs.

Her eyes looked to me. *What happens now?* To deal with our fears, we must tread lightly at first. "Just the next best step" I thought to myself as I reached for the tub closest to me. It had a blue lid, slightly battered from being shoved into trunks and stuffed under beds for years. "Let's just start here," I smiled.

One envelope after another, we waded through the papers inside. We sorted stacks of bills by ailment or issue, which pieced together a story of medical gaslighting throughout her twenties. Overdue bills that had eventually been paid were bundled together. There was shame held together with worn rubber bands and short emails with long handwritten notes from doctors' visits that yielded incomplete test results; it was all here. It was all around us, in tub after tub.

We sorted by type and looked for relief—the answers to inconclusive medical tests from a decade earlier had eventually been found and the invoices finally settled. *Phew.* She could shred these now. This chapter of Sara's life had weighed on her for so long that it seemed surprising to her that she could be free of it. The corners of her lips curled upward along with the rising pile of empty bins.

She had collected nearly two decades of bank statements and every financial notice she had ever received because she had experienced health and credit problems at one point, which then grew into lifelong shame around money. She kept every statement in case a creditor called, even though she had worked hard for years to pay back all her debts and loans. Sara viewed the paperwork warily, and when I found one form indicating that a loan had been fully paid, I suggested we should hold it up. "Let's celebrate this! You worked so hard!" I said. This mountain of account statements did not define her, and her decluttered future was just beginning.

Being able to voice the narrative of this part of her life and see, on the papers, that she had found resolution gave Sara the confidence to start shredding item after item. As the recycling bags filled up with paper confetti, Sara regained her floor space and some confidence that had been hiding in those tubs for much too long.

Underlying Issues

Burnout. Long COVID. Autoimmune diseases. Stress. Strife. Illnesses and ailments and symptoms and syndromes pile up all around like a never-ending laundry basket of socks with no matches in sight. Sometimes it can be just as hard to figure out why you don't feel well as it is to figure out why your house is so messy.

Healthy used to mean being free from disease or illness, but even the World Health Organization (WHO) updated its definition recently to include "a state of complete physical, mental and social well-being." I can tell you that none of my organizing clients have ever reached out from a state of complete well-being. Sometimes they know already why they don't feel well, and other times we must dig a little bit—through those stacks of papers and unaddressed health concerns—to sort out what is really wrong.

When we do this, we are looking for clues to follow along two pathways: how the clutter around us may be impacting our health and how our state of health (or lack thereof) influences the clutter itself. There can be a lot of reasons why this bidirectional relationship (something that takes place in two usually opposite directions) develops, and it shows up differently depending on many circumstances. Most of those reasons can be categorized into one of these two groups.

- **Direct causes:** These are things that can explicitly influence a situation, like an Amazon Prime membership, which allows lots of items to easily be delivered, or an illness that makes putting things away difficult. The membership and the illness both directly influence the volume of items around you.
- **Indirect causes:** These are facets of life less easily seen, yet they still influence a situation, like growing up with a parent who had hoarding behavior or having an unequal distribution of household labor. These behaviors influence your feelings around clutter and your available time to manage it.

The different levels of impact clutter will take in someone's life will depend on which causes he or she experiences and how he or she responds to them. These overlapping outcomes can show up and be seen in factors like volume (clutter) or consistency (days of stress felt) or strength (feeling completely overwhelmed vs just mildly annoyed).

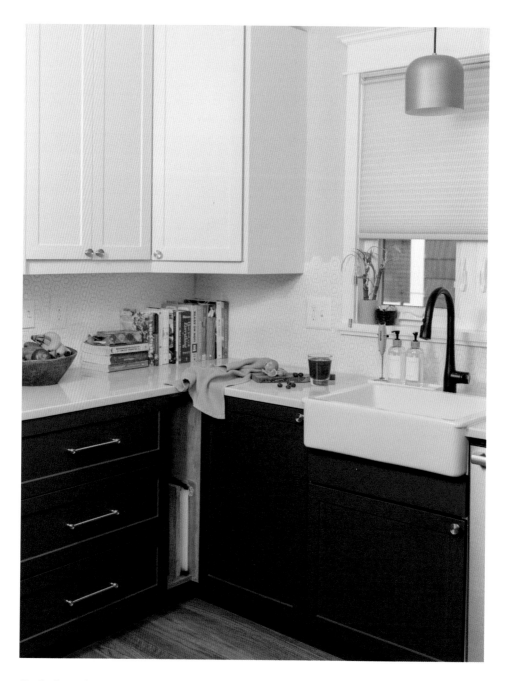

You don't need to point to each pill bottle or stack of paper around you and label them as direct or indirect causes but keep these ideas in mind while reading this book. We are going to talk a lot about ways to be more mindful in our lives, and using decluttering as a tool starts with broadening awareness of our everyday experiences. Broadening awareness is important to do because if we can better understand how health problems are showing up in our piles of clutter, we'll have more information available to make better educated decisions on what we can do to feel better.

Knowing that clutter and health issues are tangled up may cause you to feel frustrated at first—it would be so nice and easy if we were just decluttering linen closets, right? Why does it even matter if we figure out if a health issue is a function of or caused by clutter? Because I don't want you to waste your time. Or your energy. Or compromise your health anymore.

Doing some work *now* to figure out where your clutter problems stem from helps better align your actions *later* toward addressing the things that are most related to your underlying issues. For instance, if you are concerned about the volume of things in your home, then the next best step to take can be the reduction of things. And if we know that any action you take is affected by attention related challenges, then our next best step is structuring your steps with that in mind.

Laboratory-level studies on clutter and health may not be practical but that doesn't mean this is an unexamined field. In my research about clutter and health, it's been easy to find evidence that clutter in one's living space becomes connected to negative emotions and may predict high procrastination scores. And studies showing people who described their homes as cluttered were more likely to have cortisol levels associated with adverse health outcomes back up what I've seen with so many clients. Available studies tend to focus on correlated or confounding factors (situations where we cannot determine whether or not it is only clutter causing a health response) instead causation since real-world situations contain multiple sources of input.

Studies and articles are good to have as background information when examining an issue like clutter from a public health perspective, but I think we all want to know what's next. How can we take this knowledge and let it catalyze us into transforming our lives? Let's start to pull our personal stories together now to mindfully organize some of our health concerns and see what needs to be decluttered.

❖

"What do you think this is?" my client Alicia asked, picking up a single oval-shaped pill from her closet floor. An imprint of numbers and letters were on its side, so a quick Google Images search revealed it to be a wayward Klonopin, a tranquilizer resting among the carpet fibers. Thinking of the family dogs roaming around the house, I was glad we found it first.

And then Alicia popped it in her mouth.

Decluttering can be stressful for some people, but until then, I hadn't imagined people needing to medicate themselves to get through sessions with me. To be fair, she hadn't yet disclosed her medical history to me or which medications she took, so I didn't really know how this seemingly casual pill popping fit into her daily routine. Maybe it would take the edge off so she would feel more confident making decisions? Or would it numb her too much to really process what we were doing? I knew that the clutter in Alicia's home was bringing her stress—when she hired me, she was excited to have help tackling areas of her home that she had been avoiding for years—but now I started to wonder if avoidance and stress should become a bigger part of our discussions.

The Two Categories of Clutter

Clutter (n.)—a collection of disorganized or unwanted/unused/unloved items in one place; a state of confusion. *Clutter* also exists as a verb, as in the creation of that type of collection of things. Mostly, though, people use it to talk about stuff, specifically when there is too much stuff. Importantly it can also refer to the muddled nature of a task that hasn't been thought through. In this section, we'll explore some common underlying health issues connected to clutter. Underlying issues are problems, usually hidden or unknown to others, that affect an individual negatively. They are often hidden under many layers of emotions and other mental processes, which makes them hard to be seen by a casual onlooker. Of course, they can also be more visible if you know where to look, such as noticing how stress shows up in our bodies.

This isn't meant to be an exhaustive list, but I hope that you can see elements of your own life—or those of people you know—show up in the following categories. Here I will group the underlying issues I have seen most working with people to manage their clutter into two broad categories: the brain and the environment. Of course, these can overlap and are not mutually exclusive, but by naming and digging into these two, we can raise our empathy and broaden our awareness about the reasons behind the clutter. This awareness can help us decide which actions will lead to impactful results for different types of clutter.

The Brain

One of the major terms the National Association of Productivity & Organizing Professionals (NAPO) uses to discuss underlying conditions related to clutter is **brain-based conditions** (**BBCs**). They refer to these as "anything that causes a person to have ongoing difficulty or challenging differences with cognition, emotion, socialization, or behavior." It is not a diagnostic term but rather one that allows some extra focus on a specific set of conditions that will impact a person's organization or productivity. Some common examples of BBCs include:

- attention deficit hyperactivity disorder (ADHD)
- learning disabilities
- acquired brain injury (e.g., stroke) or traumatic brain injury (e.g., concussion)
- schizophrenia or other psychotic or dissociative disorders
- anxiety, depressive, or bipolar disorders
- obsessive-compulsive and related disorders, including hoarding
- intellectual disability or giftedness
- autism
- substance use disorders
- personality disorders
- post-traumatic stress disorder or other stress- or trauma-related disorders
- emotional or cognitive struggles due to physical conditions (e.g., chronic pain, menopause, thyroid disorder, narcolepsy, dementia) or medication side effects

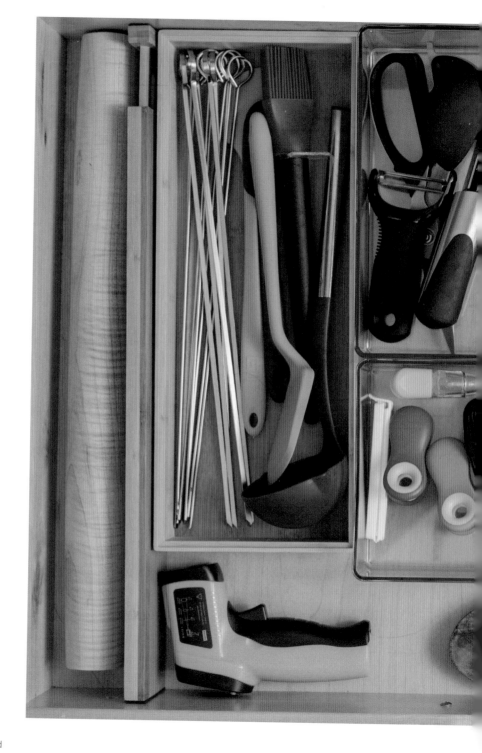

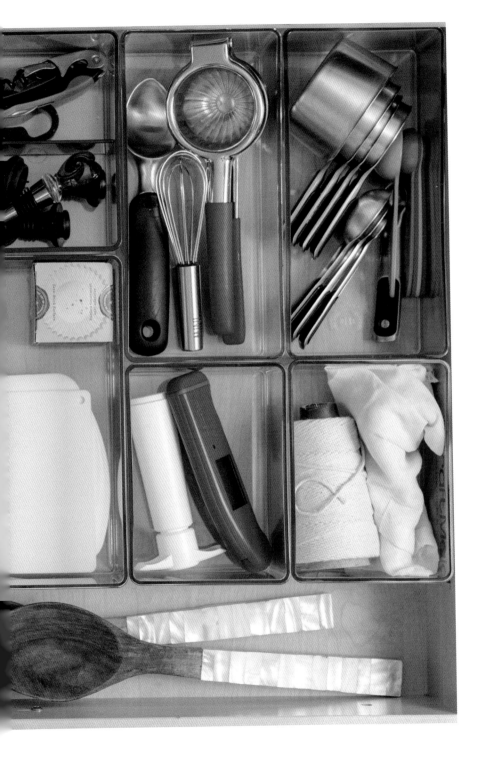

- emotional or cognitive struggles due to life circumstances (e.g., housing instability, job insecurity, abusive relationships, bereavement)

Of note, chronic illness conditions like those referenced above with "physical conditions" are important to keep in mind while unpacking issues around clutter. Chronic illness usually refers to a condition that endures for at least a year and requires ongoing medical care or consistently limits the scope of a person's daily activities. Mental health disorders like depression are one example of increasingly common chronic conditions to be aware of for this discussion.

Challenges with clutter associated with these conditions can arise due to biological conditions, like genetics and brain chemistry, or personal experiences, like trauma or abuse. Let's get into a few of these in more detail so we can be aware of their potential for impact on our clutter experiences. We will also start introducing some ways to unpack and address any concerns that might arise when you recognize a confounding situation arise between a health concern and clutter.

Executive Functioning

Brain-based conditions influence executive functioning skills, which are cognitive processes in our brain that help us do things like complete tasks and meet goals. Decluttering and managing health conditions (such as scheduling appointments or following prescriptions) are examples of tasks that require executive functioning. People with executive functioning challenges are more likely to experience challenges dealing with clutter than people who don't live with these conditions. This may happen because of sensory issues, schedule management, or the inability to focus and complete tasks.

Neurodiversity is the concept that humans vary in terms of neurocognitive ability. Everyone has both talents and weaknesses, of course, and these things vary from person to person. Attention deficit hyperactivity disorder (ADHD) is a chronic condition and type of neurodivergence that affects millions of people. ADHD includes a combination of persistent problems, such as difficulty sustaining attention, hyperactivity, and impulsive behavior. People with ADHD may also experience hyperfocus at times, which can manifest in obsessive cleaning or organizing and is often focused on a very specific subcategory of items, like becoming consumed with organizing office supplies in containers amid a room incredibly full of things they do not use or want. With a rise in adult diagnoses for ADHD in recent years, thankfully more people are getting linked with treatment and support options. At the time of writing, though, in 2023, the United States was experiencing a shortage of ADHD medications, which is a problem because they help people focus on completing tasks. Studies show that these medications work by increasing cognitive motivation: they help the person taking the medication to feel increased benefits while performing a demanding task, and at the same time, the perceived costs or struggles with completing that task are reduced. If needed, medication can be helpful for those struggling with clutter and these underlying issues. Cognitive motivation can also be supported through coaching or body-doubling situations (where people do tasks separately but in the company of others such as through online groups).

Although ADHD is not the only example of neurodiversity or brain-based challenges to take note of, I talk about it here more than others because its symptoms represent many of the underlying issues of executive function we want to pull out of this book. Executive function challenges related to clutter can manifest as struggles paying attention, categorizing items within clutter piles, and making decisions about what to declutter.

The inverse of viewing these symptoms as challenges is that sometimes they promote expansive thinking, creativity, and new directions for how to proceed in life. For instance, when sorting photographs with one client who lives with ADHD, each batch she brought forth from storage presented a new opportunity to reflect and wander through the memories they brought back. She relished these nostalgic moments and enjoyed creating albums as part of her decluttering journey. This diversity of response to stressful situations is not something that needs to be shamed. But we do want to become mindfully aware of how executive functioning appears in our lives and then see if there are practical, compassionate ways to align our skills to our desired goals.

Trauma

I've often been in my clients' underwear drawers before I've heard the specifics of their traumatic experiences.

I don't always meet the parents, partners, or children of my clients, but I feel their presence. I hear the stories.

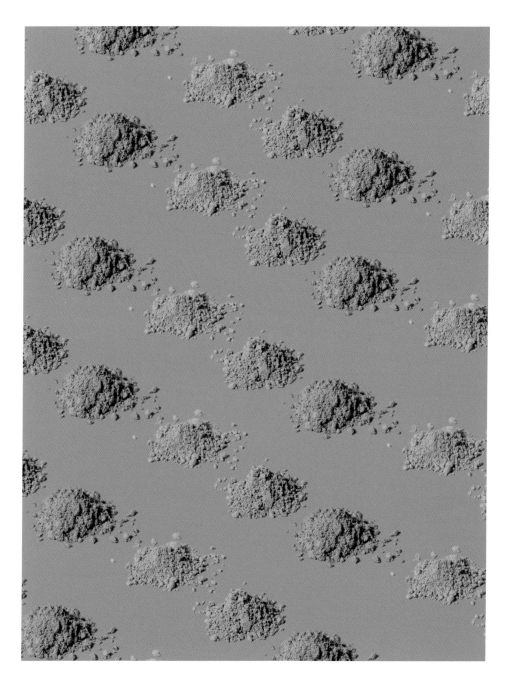

Writing this book has pushed me to face my clients' traumas in a deeper way than I have before. In person, I can sit next to them, hold a hand, pass a tissue, gently check in about appointments with their therapists. But here, in words, I need to be clear that true healing and transformation can only happen when we address underlying and presenting issues (clutter) together in a unified way. Many people say, "I should be able to do this," as we work on decluttering tasks, even though the experience of living through traumatic events has caused a struggle to complete those tasks. Removing internalized "should" statements from the vocabulary of people I work with is a long-term goal of mine.

Trauma is an emotional response to a distressing event or series of events (accidents, violence, natural disasters, for instance). The intensity and type of response will vary from person to person based on many conditions (severity, proximity, support, etc.). An ongoing situation, like growing up in a home consumed with clutter or hoarding behavior, can result in complex post-traumatic stress disorder (c-PTSD) because it may present as a series of regular and repetitive traumatic events to the person affected. Our bodies will store this trauma. The prefrontal cortex of the brain is affected significantly by trauma, and this is the part of the brain that manages executive functioning.

One manifestation of how this might appear with clutter includes the accumulation of items that may provide a protective feeling as a response to the traumatic event(s). This accumulation provides a physical barrier against the negative emotions associated with the trauma. If prompted to declutter their spaces, a stress response may be triggered for that person which in turn makes it extremely hard to call on executive skills to manage the situation because their emotions have been taken over in that moment. The prefrontal cortex is activated negatively in this moment.

Ruth Ozeki's award-winning novel *The Book of Form and Emptiness* is remarkable for its prose, for sure, but for me, I read it as a reflection of how trauma appears in some of my clients' homes. The situations described in the book are not often portrayed with compassion in popular culture. Ozeki's book is a story of a widow bringing things into her home to fill a void. Her house has begun to close in around her and her son due to this accumulation after the untimely death of her husband. Her hoarding behavior began as a way to feel safe after that traumatic event. The trauma arc displayed in the book parallels situations in real life that may start off with purchasing things or being unable to let items go, but it crescendos into mental health challenges and physical safety concerns. The visit from Child Protective Services in this book is a lightning bolt for the mother to address her clutter as a way to heal herself and her son. A gifted writer, Ozeki draws out the underlying shame and sadness the family feels—and the mother's executive functioning challenges—while cultivating empathy in the reader. For those of us who live with or care for people in similar situations, reading stories like this may make us feel less alone, less ashamed about the cluttered homes we walk among.

Emotionally regulating the prefrontal cortex in different ways helps people cope with trauma when dealing with clutter. This becomes achievable when we can bring self-awareness to which emotions we are feeling, how we are breathing, and by remaining open to our responses. Spending time in mindful awareness, without passing judgment, leads to feelings of greater emotional safety. In many of my decluttering sessions, we practice this type of emotional regulation, even without naming it, just by being mindful of our discussion, where validation and support are key tenets and making sure that the pace and tone of how we work allows for deep breathing. Holding space like this widens the window of opportunity for regulated responses to stressful situations, such as living around clutter and navigating the impact of trauma.

There is another side of trauma that is important to consider with clutter as well: what it can do to our ability to speak up for ourselves and feel confident making decisions. Making decisions confidently (and being able to act on them) is an executive functioning skill, but growing up in a home where you might not have been listened to can lead to doubt about the ability to do this. A seventy-year-old retired military executive client I work with still remembers his mother not allowing him to make decisions about where to put his things as a child, and he connects that to his own uncertainty when trying to declutter to this day.

The trauma of not being listened to may also show up as an inability to feel worthy of love or money or other nice things. This lack and unworthiness may drive us toward perfectionism, constantly seeking approval from others or always yearning toward self-improvement. My clients in this situation want regular reassurance that they are doing things right, or they are acutely focused on small and very specific decluttering tasks, like the organization of a bathroom drawer with minutia-level categorization. Distrusting our own opinions and a fear of making mistakes can lead to overconsumption of things through shopping or addictions or even ideas and actions that may be harmful. One does this by always reaching for the next recommended product or way of doing something because of a distrust that what was purchased or practiced is sufficient.

I don't want to discount asking for opinions or organizing in a way that makes you enjoy your space, but we must ask where this desire comes from, and how it shapes our decision making. The more we can recognize where this drive comes from, the less we will be controlled by it and instead remain calmly aware.

Shame and Stigma

Shame and stigma exist around clutter and metastasize internally as stress, social isolation, and rage. It may come from our relatives who don't agree with how we manage our homes, or internal shame brought on by perfectionism. Mental health and anxiety issues run very deep inside our feelings about whether or not we think we are accepted within our communities. If your community includes regularly interacting with social media, then you may see a lot of extremely organized people online and that may bring feelings of shame about the clutter that exists in your life. The stigma around having a messy home is prevalent and only exacerbated through the nonstop barrage of pretty pantries and organized closets shown online. Gendered stereotypes around the creation and maintenance of "organized" homes promote internalized shame for many women who do not perform as dictated by these antiquated and patriarchal standards. Constantly buying new sizes of baskets and containers is easier some days than fighting our inner critics.

Full disclosure: I love television, especially reality shows of the house or housewife variety (probably stemming from my early fascination with *The Real World*) so it makes sense that I have watched at least a few episodes of nearly all the shows involving decluttering and organizing—from the ones focused on extreme hoarding behavior to the ones highlighting extreme organizational systems. These dramatic transformations, or before-and-after story arcs, can be compelling, but unfortunately, they can also contribute to much of the shame and stigma that people feel around clutter and their homes. Social media and television shows present us with two options for managing clutter: you either have a highly designed and meticulously organized space or you have a hoarder's home. While these images can raise awareness of the struggles that people face and the help that decluttering can bring, the diametrically opposed options cause many people feelings of shame because they do not see themselves at the "after" level of organization. They are apt to self-identify with the "before" image only.

Shame and stigma can be strengthened or lessened depending on the ties between our self-identification and how we interact within groups. So far, we have explored health and clutter with a focus on personal challenges and self-assessments. Now it's time to recognize that as social animals, we depend on and are influenced by our social connections. We all need to feel like we belong, and when we feel like we belong, this can improve our mental and physical health. For example, aging adults benefit from group classes that bring them together over shared interests. As the impact of social media continues to be studied, research is constantly being updated about how our health can be impacted (negatively or positively) by the types of social groups we find ourselves involved with online and off.

Shame and stigma thrive on isolation and whether we see ourselves as part of a group (an "in-group") or as not identifying with a group (an "out-group"). There has been a lot of praise for and backlash to Marie Kondo in the years since her best-selling *The Life Changing Magic of Tidying Up* came out. Those of us who feel aligned with her mission and practice will be connected to the KonMari in-group mentality, and we may (at least I do) get very animated when people in an out-group, like those who say she places a limit on the number of books you should have—not true!—or that she shouldn't sell products, speak out against her.

One solution to feeling aligned to the right in-group for you is ensuring you are a part of a community-care network to help address the health and clutter concerns you have. Translating what I first learned about HIV/AIDS programs into decluttering networks has been eye opening!

HIV posttest clubs were the topic of my graduate school thesis in the early 2000s. These clubs were the one space in certain countries where people who were brave enough to go in for an HIV test could get continued support in a group setting—regardless of how they tested. This distinction was interesting because there were many support group options for people who had tested positive—and rightly so! HIV-positive people needed to get linked into care and treatment options ASAP, and these groups helped do so—but I wondered why the people who had tested negative had little support after receiving their result. They had been concerned they might have been exposed to HIV but luckily had managed to test negative at this point in time. The posttest clubs were a safe place for people to talk about their experiences, ask questions, and get advice on being able to remain negative. These clubs helped decrease the enor-

Journaling about Clutter and Our Brains

Length of Time: 15 minutes

Materials Needed: Something to write with (pen, pencil, marker) and something to write on (journal or notebook—something with enough room to write in a few times as you move through the exercises in this book)

Prompt: Move through the list of questions and write down what comes to mind without censoring yourself.

Although the promise of clearing out physical clutter is often what prompts people to reach out to a professional organizer, adding in introspection to understand and address the underlying issues will yield the most long-lasting results. In this exercise, I want to offer some space for active reflection on which underlying issues you may have, specifically around the brain-based concerns we've just discussed.

In terms of health concerns related to clutter, let's work through this like preparing for a physical exam. Many people have visited a doctor in their lives at least once and are familiar with that concept—and depending on what you get out of this exercise, you may want to bring some of these issues up with your health providers. We'll do this writing exercise to start collecting some data on which elements of our health situations are leading to negative experiences with clutter, and then later we'll discuss how to use this information to better advocate for ourselves and any changes we need to make to relieve concerns we may have.

Journaling, the practice of writing for ourselves without censoring, can help people let out feelings and experiences that have been bottled up. Let this experience be a way to relieve stress and declutter ideas and thoughts that may feel overwhelming.

During your journaling session for this writing exercise, give yourself a quiet space to write and think and spend around three minutes reflecting on each of the following questions.

1. What do you think of when you think of clutter? Have you ever felt shame around clutter?

2. What came up for you when you read the story about Sara at the start of this chapter?

3. Having read about brain-based conditions and clutter, can you think of any examples of how that shows up in people you know? How about in yourself?

4. What is a way someone struggling with health concerns around clutter could be supported by other people?

5. Is there anything else you want to write about clutter and health that I haven't asked you about yet?

Great job getting started on these exercises. We'll add to these thoughts and ideas throughout this book, so keep your notes close to you.

mous stigma around HIV and worked to end the shame around the disease. These posttest clubs helped support them on their path.

Community-care networks for clutter and health situations can and do exist. They may look like accountability hours where online people separately complete decluttering or life admin tasks, or peer support groups bonded over shared diagnoses and trading tips for illness management. There are so many ways to think about underlying issues related to health and clutter, and how to navigate them—let's take some time to put our thoughts together with this writing exercise.

The Environment

Environmental health influences on clutter can range from concerns with building materials to ease moving around a room and include categories as varied as sunlight and hoarding. For this section, we'll focus mainly on situations within the built environment, structures created by people and the features and facilities making them up and constituting the places where we live and work, with some suggested thinking on larger environmental concerns. In the next chapter, "Home," we'll dive deeper into the aesthetic factors of the built environment. Here we are focused on the functions of a space that influence our quality of life and what relation that has to clutter. Although we are looking at these features today as adult readers who typically have at least some agency over our environments, we want to also reflect on what this experience can mean for children who have less (if any) control of their built environments. The environments where children grow up can set the framework for their relationship to clutter.

Hoarding

Mental health conditions do not typically get their own television shows, aside from the problematic spring 2023 season of *Vanderpump Rules*, but hoarding disorder has been the exception. Hoarding disorder is an ongoing difficulty of throwing away or parting with possessions because you believe that you need to save them. Hoarding behaviors can come out through the accumulation of large volumes of items, regardless of their financial value, and is tied to significant stress when faced with decluttering.

Hoarding behavior is not just stressful for the person dealing with the condition; it can also be physically and emotionally unhealthy for other people living in the home, especially children. Children who experience the stress of hoarding are living in a traumatic environment and are therefore dealing with the impact that carries. In her book *I'm Glad My Mom Died*, Jennette McCurdy shares that her mother was a hoarder. After being diagnosed with stage-four breast cancer—when McCurdy herself was only two years old—her mother started hoarding. "My grandparents moved in with us during my mother's illness, and my mother, as a result of her cancer, she became a hoarder," McCurdy said. "Because she was so close to seeing her fate, she suddenly attached meaning and significance to the tiny—I mean she'd say, 'Well, you touched that Kleenex, so I need it.'" Throughout her memoir McCurdy shares how this living experience affected her from childhood and into adulthood.

Clutter buildup and hoarding are a form of numbing against the things you are afraid of facing or are dealing with. They appear as traumatic experiences in the brain for people living in these environments. Unfortunately, mental health services are underfunded and hard to access throughout parts of the United States and elsewhere. With a growing elderly population, it is expected that hoarding situations are expected to increase in the coming years. If clutter and hoarding problems were able to be more widely recognized and their treatment supported under health insurance plans or state service funding opportunities, then more children would not grow up in houses with these types of issues, and adults with mental health problems would be better served.

Adults I work with who come from childhoods spent in homes exhibiting hoarding behavior often face a complicated path in life when they are trying to make a home for themselves. They may remember the hoarding situations of their childhoods and don't want to live like that, but choosing a new path means breaking away from family norms. If a hoarding environment is what you know, you may find a sense of safety and familiarity with it, even as you understand that it could be unhealthy. People often seize on a transition moment—a job change, a new baby or trying to get pregnant, a move, and so on—to try to make this change, as though a transition offers permission for a different future. This allows the onus of the decision (to declutter) to be on the external factor (the move, job, baby) as opposed to an internal change in value or dynamics (from how their family of origin dealt with clutter).

Beyond Our Walls

Beyond the walls of our homes or buildings where we work and spend our time, there are environmental health factors that may influence our relationship with clutter. These are situations that are likely outside our immediate and personal sphere of control. These are things to be aware of so we can consider how broader policy and structural impact may be needed.

Depending on our income and various factors that influence where we live, many aspects of the physical environment are outside of our direct control, unless we consider—and get involved with—how political decisions impact our domestic space. You might be wondering how this relates to clutter: it does by prioritizing community health and well-being, which also influence habits and actions around how we purchase, accumulate, share, or reduce stuff. Some opportunities to declutter in our lives happen within our medicine cabinets and it is great to spend time on activities like that, just as it is beneficial to sometimes investigate advocating for broader structural decluttering. Here are some examples of policies and movements to be aware of beyond your walls:

- **Spatial justice.** Spatial justice links social justice to space and is a field that analyzes the impact of regional planning and urban planning decisions. Spatial justice work will examine whether or not a home is within walkable distance to a safe public park, for example, which will increase opportunity for movement, fresh air and sunlight to those living around it. Conversely, a home surrounded by heavy automobile traffic, or industrial facilities releasing harmful chemicals means a likely uptick in air or water borne contaminants that can directly lead to health issues. Currently there are countless examples of neighborhoods uniting to protect open space from development or ensuring their public-school parks are not shut down by the city, thus shaping the larger physical environment surrounding their homes.

- **Affordable/safe housing.** It's hard to even consider the idea of a healthy decluttered home if you don't feel safe there. Let's start with the idea that for most people, homes are intended to provide a sense of security and stability yet there are many people who do not feel good or safe in their homes, often because they *aren't* safe. One major structural obstacle within this category is redlining, and it has already shaped many neighborhoods in discriminatory ways. If people have been subject to abuse or predatory lending where they are worried every day about paying for their space, stress can accumulate.

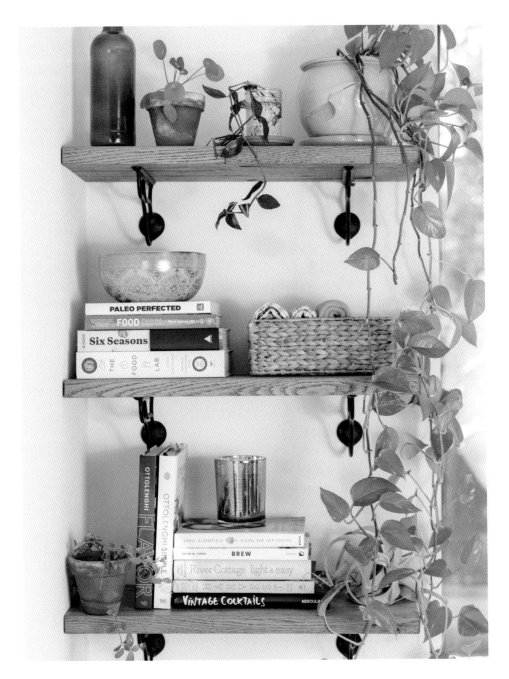

- **Food deserts.** When people live in areas where they do not have ready access to affordable, safe, and healthy options for food and basic household supplies their health will be affected. Nutritional, cognitive, and chronic conditions can arise in these situations. If the only or least costly options for household shopping are with stores that sell large quantities of items people run the risk of purchasing more than they can use and store before things expire or create unmanageable clutter in their homes.

Although this book does not go into detail on all of these nuanced and important topics of environmental health concerns, consider keeping them in mind as you declutter your world and experience the joy that comes from a functional, soothing space—you may be inspired to help declutter on a larger scale. We do not have to choose which of these actions are most important. Being compassionate allows us to understand that multiple issues can intersect and be relevant at the same time. We may also want to address them at different times and in different ways. Some days you may focus on your personal environmental health concerns—making sure the filters in your air purifier are changed—and other days you may read up on local housing-development laws in your town to see who you want to support for office. All these things together help lead us toward improved health situations and decluttered environments, which will enhance life overall.

Introspection for this section comes down to this:

- Do you have the ability to decide on the environment in which you live?
- Do you have the agency to affect change for yourself or for others?
- If you have this agency how can you protect your space from clutter and health issues?

Imagine order in your built environment as the platform on which you can spend your life doing what is most meaningful for you, which includes having a space that aligns with your needs and lifestyle. This is why considering the big picture of health and built environments of people is vital; it's also why holistic assessments of health need to consider how the built environment influences every person's relationship to objects, spaces, and each other.

Luckily, an entire field is dedicated to this: medical (or health) sociology. Medical sociology examines the structural components that influence health. It can also be defined as the scientific study of the social patterning of health. It considers how social factors, such as class, race, gender, religion, ethnicity, kinship networks, marriage, educational status, age, place, and cultural practices, influence human health. In the interest of removing some of the shame and health conditions associated with clutter at home on the individual level, it helps to remember that our experiences are shaped by the larger world beyond our walls.

While thinking broadly about these intersected concerns, you must know where to direct your attention if you want to change your situation. Do your problems with clutter stem from a biomedical issue, like not getting enough sleep, which makes it hard to complete tasks at home? Is it a behavioral issue, like a husband never putting his clothes away? Or is it a structural issue, like not having the opportunity to live in a home with safe conditions and storage options? Most likely it's a combination of these things, but at any given point, it's helpful to take a deep breath and assess what the main driver of your feeling of being overwhelmed is and think about ways you can improve the situation.

WRITING EXERCISE

The Environmental Assessment

Time Needed: 15 minutes

Materials Needed: Journal or notebook (wherever you started writing earlier) and a pen/pencil/marker

Prompt: Be mindful of what external factors show up in our environments that can change our health clutter. Answer the following questions:

1. How do you feel in the environments where you spend time?

2. Are there any biomedical factors influencing clutter in your home?

3. Are there any behavioral factors influencing clutter in your life?

4. Are there any structural issues influencing your relationship with clutter?

5. Is there anything else about environmental health you think is important to connect to your experience with clutter?

6. What feels like it is within your control to address?

7. How do social factors relate to clutter in your life? Have you seen this anywhere?

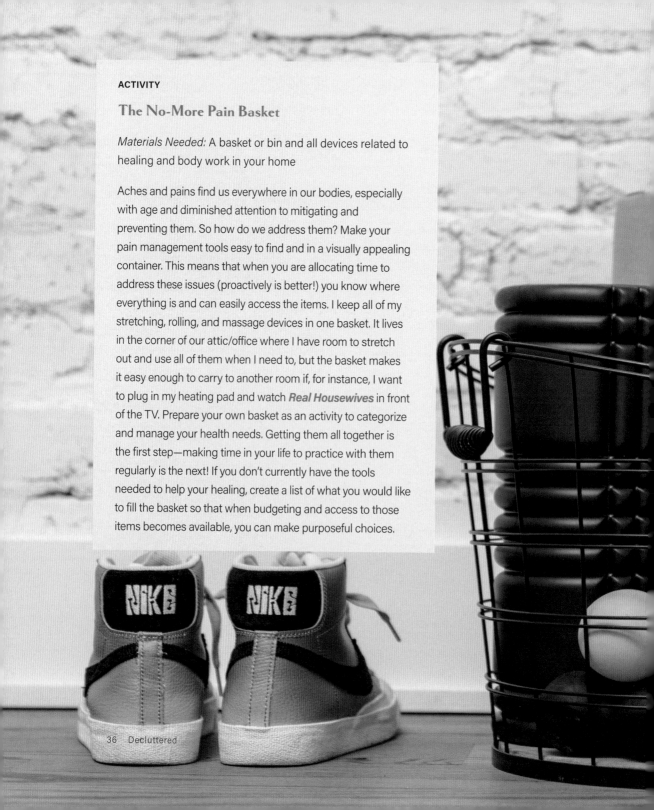

ACTIVITY

The No-More Pain Basket

Materials Needed: A basket or bin and all devices related to healing and body work in your home

Aches and pains find us everywhere in our bodies, especially with age and diminished attention to mitigating and preventing them. So how do we address them? Make your pain management tools easy to find and in a visually appealing container. This means that when you are allocating time to address these issues (proactively is better!) you know where everything is and can easily access the items. I keep all of my stretching, rolling, and massage devices in one basket. It lives in the corner of our attic/office where I have room to stretch out and use all of them when I need to, but the basket makes it easy enough to carry to another room if, for instance, I want to plug in my heating pad and watch *Real Housewives* in front of the TV. Prepare your own basket as an activity to categorize and manage your health needs. Getting them all together is the first step—making time in your life to practice with them regularly is the next! If you don't currently have the tools needed to help your healing, create a list of what you would like to fill the basket so that when budgeting and access to those items becomes available, you can make purposeful choices.

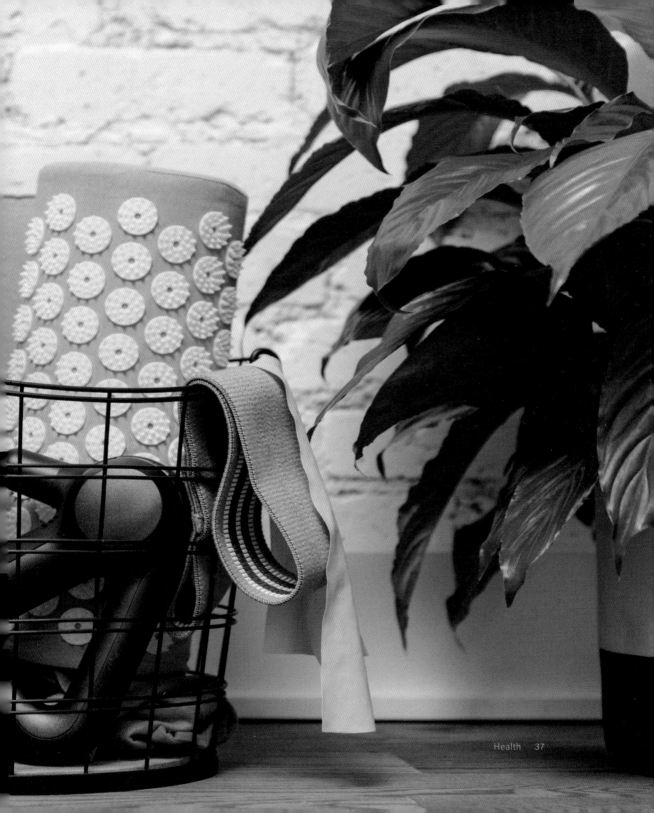

Decluttering Our Health: How to Take the Next Step

With this nuanced background information on the underlying issues related to clutter, you might feel your stress levels staring to rise. Sorry about that! I certainly don't intend to leave you feeling overwhelmed, but it is important that we start with noticing. We need to notice how ideas or concepts show up in our bodies (sometimes as headaches or neck pain for instance) and not judge ourselves for having reactions. With this noticing, we can start to declutter differently, more mindfully.

Mindfulness

What is mindfulness, and why does it matter to your health? Mindfulness is really just paying attention to the present moment without judgment. It's about connecting with ourselves and others authentically. Mindfulness practices can take many shapes—meditation, breathing techniques, and more—with a common theme of allowing our nervous systems to relax and our minds to get quieter. Earlier we discussed activated states of the brain when under distress, especially with challenges of executive functioning. Mindfulness helps regulate these emotions and that state of being, principally so that our prefrontal cortex operates well.

People can experience mindful moments doing many things since there are lots of ways we can be fully present and experience these moments of quiet contemplation in our lives. Unfortunately, that just isn't a state that many of us live in often, which is too bad since mindfulness has many so different benefits. Regular mindfulness practices can help us with the following.

- **Physical:** lowered blood pressure, improved heart health, stronger immune response, improved sleep
- **Mental:** improved attention, greater creativity, better memory, reduced bias
- **Emotional:** greater stress resilience, improved mood, reduced anxiety and depression, greater empathy
- **Behavioral:** less reactivity, greater persistence, more ethical behavior, greater patience

The key here is that the more we experience these moments—the more we allow ourselves to fully embody a quiet, contemplative state—the more our brains get to benefit and adapt over time. This adaptation is called neuroplasticity. Neuroplasticity is when the brain changes or forms new neural connections. These new connections, built through practicing mindfulness, calm the amygdala and your prefrontal cortex, which brings us back to the underlying brain conditions we discussed earlier. This type of neuroplasticity also occurs when we regularize new habits toward our decluttering goals. Quite literally we are decluttering stressed out connections in our brains to prioritize new, healthy ones aligned to our priorities.

Remember that many of the brain-based conditions have an impact on, or are affected by, challenges within our prefrontal cortex. Consistent mindfulness practices can help us regulate and promote resilience within our brains. Mindfulness trains you not to get overtaken by strong emotions too quickly and helps you recover from distress more easily. Regarding clutter, this distress can show up as being incredibly overwhelmed by piles of things or when a person with hoarding behavior is asked to discard some items.

Mindfulness can also help you maintain composure during crises while also reducing inflammation and the impact of chronic stress on the body. It does this by expanding what some people call your "window of tolerance," which is the space between too much arousal (perhaps from a triggering event, like an upended laundry basket in the hallway) and too little arousal (a restful state, like the moment before you walked upstairs to see the basket). Within this window is a middle ground that offers a neutral opportunity to react to the event. With more practice and greater awareness of being in this zone, you are better able to practice empathy and use perspective to lead to compassionate responses. One client who practiced mindfulness with me was able to reduce her outbursts at her children when confronted with toys not put away. Having taught herself to take three slow breaths whenever entering the playroom, she had just enough extra time to get into her window of tolerance zone and give a response focused on encouragement and not rage.

When stress and trauma shrink your window of tolerance, maintaining stability in your work/life rhythms becomes difficult, but mindfulness allows us to widen a window of tolerance to improve our compassionate responses. It also gives our executive functioning skills more of a chance to work. The more ingrained mindfulness practice becomes in your life, the deeper its impact will be so that when you are presented with challenges, you will be able to address them clearly and without reactivity. You don't need a lot of time to add this benefit into your life; even five minutes a day is helpful. Regularizing a habit like this, making it a part of your everyday life, is what will bring you results and move you from thinking of it as something you should do to something that is simply a part of how you live. Just another next best step to try.

As this becomes a regular part of your routine, you'll want to consider the awareness around clutter in your life with the same sort of mindfulness—you are aware of it, but are you removing judgment from it? This is more easily started with the sorts of regularly occurring clutter most people experience at some point: a stack of mail or dishes on a counter that haven't been put away. Can you exist around this type of clutter without associating a meaning to it? Depending on your window of tolerance, this could be difficult or easy for you.

Mindful organizing brings together an awareness of health and clutter concerns—this showed up in your earlier responses to the writing exercise—and offers time and space to increase our window of tolerance and calm the nervous system. This then allows us to mitigate the impact clutter can have on our health.

The World Health Organization (WHO) says that mental health is a state of well-being in which the individual realizes his or her own abilities, can cope with the normal stresses of life, can work productively and fruitfully, and is able to make a contribution to his or her community. When our emotional, psychological, and social well-being is unbalanced, we suffer. And mental health challenges are often confounding situations for managing clutter. That's why I'm always glad to hear when my clients schedule our sessions just before their therapy sessions—because they know that facing the personal stories packed within their homes will unearth significant feelings and that processing them with their trusted mental health professionals is a good complementary step to the decluttering work.

Once we have a sense of what health areas may be of concern, we also want to understand the magnitude of the problem. This means we need data. What we are trying to do is get enough data (qualitative and quantitative) to steer us toward the areas that need attention. Triangulating the data means using different methods to collect and analyze information from different sources to get what is hopefully a robust answer. Public health programs and policies use data to advocate for funding and support. You can use data to advocate for your health too. No single measurement (for example, number of loads of laundry done per week) equates to a whole answer, but we do need some data points in order to choose impactful actions to take to get more lasting decluttered lives.

Setting a Goal to Declutter for Health

Time Needed: 20 minutes

Materials Needed: Journal or notebook (wherever you started writing earlier) and a pen/pencil/marker

Prompt: Now it's time to identify specific goals and then act on decluttering your health. Without goals, how can we know if we are moving in the right direction? This is a two-part prompt that will help you develop a specific goal and visualize how it feels when you reach that milestone.

First, take five minutes to set a vision, intention, or goal. What aspect of your health has most come to mind while reading this chapter and working through the previous exercises? How have you thought about the bidirectional relationship clutter has with your health? I'll provide some examples. The following are some statements you can use to begin your answers.

- A vision: an aspiration for the future ("I am decluttered.")

- An intention: a guiding principle for how you want to live ("I will declutter regularly.")

- A goal: a desired result ("I am able to declutter without stress.")

The vision, intentions, and goals you set around health and clutter will be varied and personal—as they pertain to your priorities. Once we know what these are, decluttering things that do not help direct energy toward your goals becomes easier. The more clearly you can articulate your answers to the above statements and the more often you reflect on them, the more likely you are to see changes in your behavior and feelings. We are writing or speaking or thinking these out to help support you on your journey to decluttering your health.

Now we are ready for more detail with setting our goals.

Second prompt: It's time to focus on what makes you feel your best. Consider the following questions and without censoring yourself write for at least ten minutes about what comes to mind.

- How would you like to feel?

- When do you feel your best?

- What would you like to see?

- What smells bring you peace?

- Where do you feel calm?

- What sounds cultivate positive feelings for you?

- What is nonnegotiable for your health?

Reflect on your notes here to see how your desires around feeling good align with your goals focused on decluttering. Let these messages influence decisions you make for your attention and energy, and consider how these relate to what you learned from doing the environmental assessment earlier.

From Goals to Action

Moving from awareness to action may come as quickly as tossing an apple core in the trash or as slowly as swimming through a dumpster full of donated clothing. What is your trip wire (a passive triggering mechanism or moment) that changes a behavior or action? How bad does it have to get before you want a change? Are a few pieces of clothing on a bench fine but not so many that they overflow? Is a half-full laundry basket fine? But when it's full, do you start a load? For one of my clients, their benchmark to deal with clutter was every time they couldn't close a drawer in their kitchen. You can come up with whatever feels right if you are able to name and see it. You can use your trip wire to push you to check in and change what's going on.

Because this book aims to look at clutter through different lenses (under the examination of health, home, and beyond), it provides a holistic model that can help you work toward stronger findings, answers, and clarity on what support you will need for long-lasting changes. Identifying your points for movement and acting on concerns you have identified is a piece of this model.

Sara's story earlier in this chapter stands as a cautionary tale of how problems with the health care system can lead to clutter, which exacerbates anxiety and shame. Early on in life many people are taught "oh keep it, just in case," for every piece of mail received from an institution or "professional," but not every piece of paper is helpful, and certainly having ten boxes of paperwork when a current or new doctor says, "Let's go through your records together" isn't practical. With Sara, I looked at her medical files with her to pull out infrequent tests (MRIs, baseline hormone levels) that might be useful to have on hand, so we set those aside to keep, but we let go of the hundreds of statements that were just explanations of benefits (EOBs), miscellaneous Health Insurance Portability and Accountability Act (HIPPA) notices, or tests done whose results didn't yield anything specific (or which she knew she could now easily access via her online platforms). These were items clogging up her boxes and preventing her from being able to access what she really needed.

Sara had kept these papers in part because she had been told year after year, she was fine, even as her symptoms and ailments changed and complicated her life. She knew something was wrong and thought keeping all the papers would help her get the answers and treatments she really needed. Medical gaslighting is pervasive for women, especially women of color. Because women are underrepresented in medical studies and women's health concerns receive less funding for research and treatment, we often have to act as our own detectives and advocates to get to the root of medical pains and ailments. Struggling with undiagnosed and undertreated

Health Care Provider Script

Time Needed: 10 minutes at home before an appointment and then a few moments of attention with your provider

Materials Needed: Journal or notebook (wherever you started writing earlier) and a pen/pencil/marker

Prompt: Go through the list of questions and without censoring yourself write what comes to mind when you consider the relationship you have between your health and clutter. Use these questions as you assess:

- How many days last week did you feel overwhelmed by clutter?

- What are the symptoms you experience physically and emotionally when this happens?

- What unplanned changes in the amount and quality of sleep and overall changes in mental health occurred?

- What examples of biomedical, behavioral or structural conditions affecting your health are you aware of?

- How many minutes or hours were spent doing things that make you feel good, including exercise, meditation, movement, and sex?

Now that you've reflected and articulated some concrete examples of health conditions related to clutter, we have data to begin the discussion with your provider. That's great! Whenever possible, see someone whom you trust who specializes in the area you are examining. Here are some ways to begin the conversation with your provider using the data you have collected on yourself:

- I'd like to tell you about a time when I . . .

- I'm concerned that this is an example of . . .

- Here are some findings from an assessment I've done about my health (include here any relevant information about the symptoms and feelings you have been having, pulling from the self-assessments you have done in this chapter and using data if possible—blood pressure measurements, examples of when things felt off, etc.).

- I'd like to align what's going on in my health with how I would like to feel. Are you able to help me with this, or can you refer me to the right type of provider who can?

In later chapters, we'll continue this thread of drilling down into where we see clutter showing up in our lives and directing our efforts at mitigating its effects.

symptoms for many years can manifest in boxes of paperwork from every single doctor visit. Going through these boxes with Sara was like revisiting the shame and pain she had experienced for years, but getting to the root of the issue and knowing she did not have to stay tied to those stories for medical, legal, or sentimental reasons moving forward freed her from having to take these boxes on any more moves around the country.

Now that you have done an assessment of what feels cluttered within your health or how your health may be affected by clutter, consider who you need to discuss this with. If you have noticed any untended-to biological or behavioral challenges, you may want to speak to a health care provider. This is not always comfortable for people, so I've included some sample script ideas that can be modified and used to facilitate a dialogue that will prioritize your concerns.

Creativity

During high school and college, I spent a few summers working at the Children's AIDS Project (CAP) in Boston. I learned about this program while working in the Housing Department at the AIDS Action Committee. At CAP we went on field trips, played games, and offered therapy with the staff, who infused counseling with art and play for children living with HIV/AIDS. One of the best teaching moments of my early career was seeing how therapists could make tough conversations digestible and enjoyable. Drawing and writing stories about taking medications and acting out scenarios with the in-house therapist brought us all together and helped the kids manage complicated emotions.

Years later, creativity as a healing exercise appeared in my life again and reminded me of how artistic expression can and should be part of health initiatives. When I moved to the Kingdom of Swaziland in 2008, I kept myself open to seeing if I could create this type of opportunity. And in 2011, I finally did. You couldn't live in Swaziland around 2011 and not know about HIV/AIDS— at the time it had the highest prevalence in the world, and no one wasn't somehow affected. But data doesn't always translate to behavior or policy changes. Sometimes we need to feel and experience impact and stories visually and with heart.

We wanted to try something different. Working with a local gallery, we met with a dozen or so local artists. Each artist was paired with one of our President's Emergency Plan for AIDS Relief (PEPFAR) partners, organizations funded to carry out HIV/AIDS services in line with the priorities and plans set by the Government of the Kingdom of Swaziland (GKOS). The partners brought their artists to visit their programs and meet with their staff and beneficiaries; then the artists created works that told the story of those projects with respect, compassion, and solidarity. When we finished, we held an art show open to the public. People could also purchase the works directly from the artists, further supporting their creative work. This was based on an exercise I'd learned from the embassy communications person in Zambia, and I brought it to Swaziland when I moved there.

It was amazing. It had everything: tapestries woven about children in orphanages, paintings showing medicine delivered via bicycles, a larger-than-life sculpture created using sterilized forceps from the national voluntary medical male circumcision program. Collages and photography and all manners of media were used. In the story of what the HIV/AIDS epidemic was doing to the country at that time, the pieces created a way to share insights and emotions still not translatable in data tables.

This experience stays with me, even now in my decluttering journey. I wonder how we can use art and creativity to make sense of the clutter in our health story, our well-being. Are there ways to use play or beauty or creativity to help us examine, work through, and make sense of the mess around us?

Making space in your life for creative ritual is healing in and of itself. We can also center creativity as one way to explore our relationships to our homes and our objects. If you are stuck on where to begin, the following is an exercise to help. Often our lives feel cluttered and overwhelmed with basic tasks, but even then—especially then—it is important to allow space for creativity and play.

One of the most challenging parts of writing this book has been reckoning with how to describe the levels of suffering I see people face with clutter. After spending over twenty years in HIV/AIDS clinics and programs, I don't think that suffering and illnesses need to compete for my attention, because we shouldn't have a cap on our compassion. I think decluttering our lives is an important focus for wellness and well-being efforts. People don't recognize how much clutter affects their ability to achieve goals and passions, whether it comes to their physical movements or professional ambitions or creativity and rest rituals. The higher purpose of decluttering is getting

CREATIVE EXERCISE

Center Creativity

Time Needed: 20 minutes

Materials Needed: Whatever creative materials you have around or feel called to find (markers, pencils, magazines, glue, etc.)

Prompt: Start by asking yourself, "What is the story I am learning about clutter in my life?" As you process what comes up, your task is to create something that brings this forward in a new way creatively. Giving yourself these few minutes and this opportunity to process your feelings about clutter can unlock new ideas and perspectives beyond straightening up shelves or folding clothes.

Once you identify the emotional core of your idea, select a medium that speaks to you. For example, are you feeling a burst of joy that you'd love to convey via acrylic paints and collage? Or are you recognizing the residue of anger and frustration that has been hiding in your inner storage compartments and need a cathartic practice, such as writing a monologue and performing it—even to yourself—with the intention of giving yourself closure. Some media to consider are:

- photography (doesn't have to be a fancy camera, nearly every phone today takes pictures)

- collage (tangible or digital, vision boards)

- words (poetry, short stories, journaling)

- movement (dance)

- sound (singing, instruments, curating playlists)

Some of these may be materials you've come across while decluttering that have sparked an interest or an idea you'd like to bring to life.

Whatever your choice of material, spend your time expressing your answers to the question asked above to enhance what you have learned about clutter and your health. What represents this awareness? While this creation is meant just for you (if that is your preference), think about what can be created to live in your space or share with others to tell your story.

In the next chapter, we will talk more about how experiencing art, whether through viewing or creating it, can help us process emotions and regulate our nervous systems. Doing this in connection with your decluttering experience can help infuse deeper growth along your path of mindful organizing.

unstuck from whatever is weighing us down emotionally and physically by removing it from our lives. It may be scary, but it's ultimately worth it.

There's a powerful connection between our homes and our health. When we're surrounded by clutter, we feel the weight of that clutter inside ourselves. Similarly, when we feel stressed and overwhelmed, our environments often reflect that inner imbalance. Because our internal and external experiences are directly connected, the powerful truth is that when we change one, we change the other.

When we minimize clutter and eliminate anything we don't need, love, or value in our environments, we establish a foundation for awareness, calm, and ease. As we peel away the layers and begin to establish new systems of order, we also assess and adjust outdated habits and patterns that cause stress and disorder. By approaching organization holistically, we create a foundation for healthy, balanced, and peaceful living.

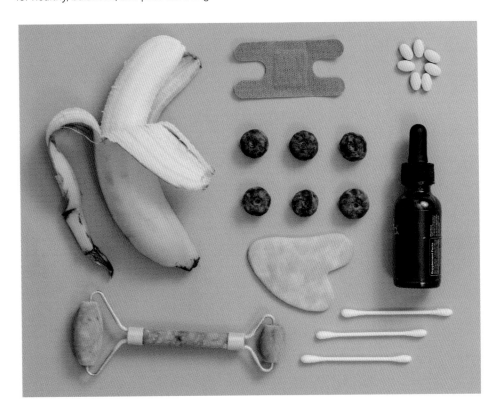

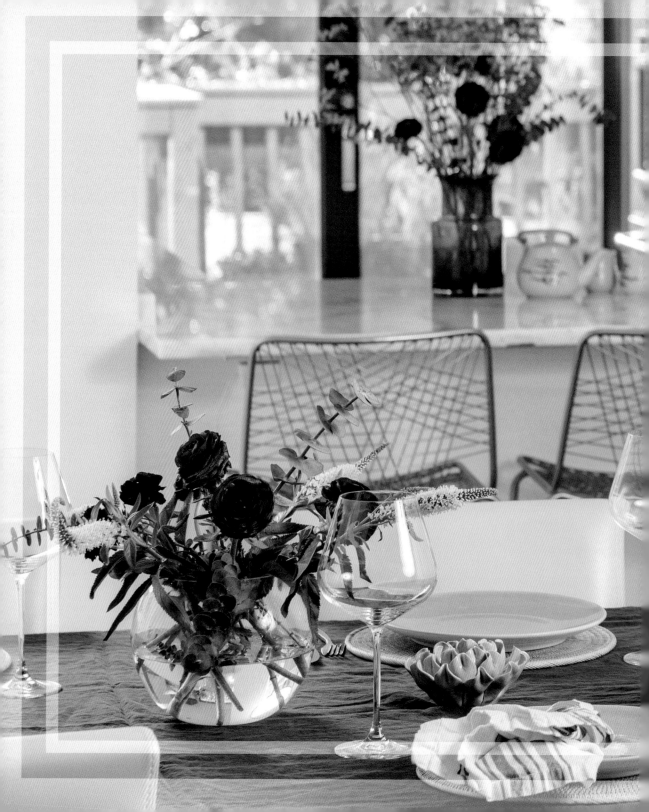

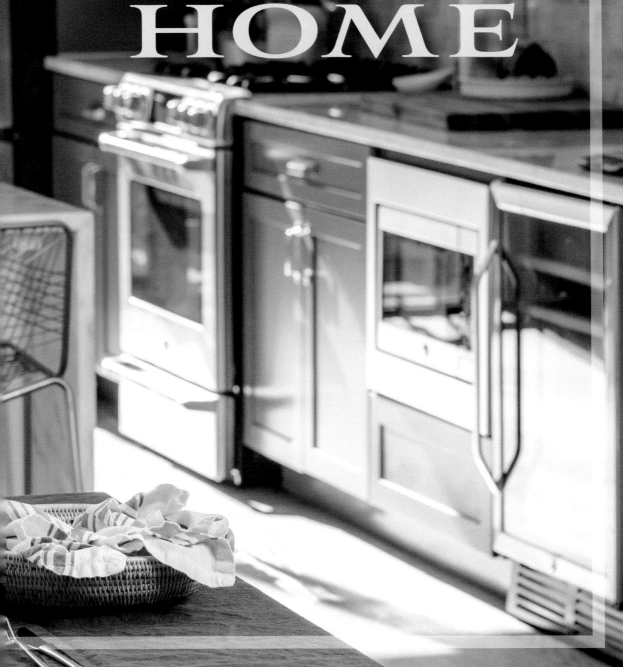

HOME

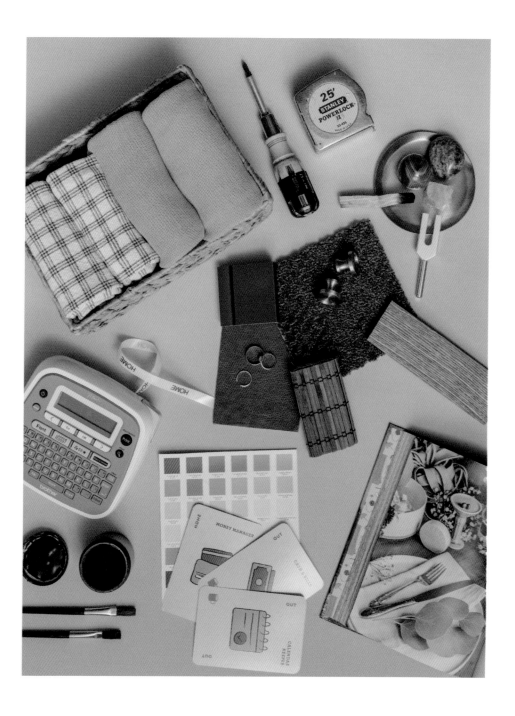

HOME

Her house was just two blocks from mine, but when I walked inside, I felt transported to another land. Stacks of magazines were piled high against the wall of what I guessed was a dining room, primarily because I spotted a long oval-shaped wooden table beneath all the clothing. Laundry? Donations? It probably didn't have a purpose or destination. There was little reason to be found in the room, least of all among the clutter.

Shyly, Beth invited me inside. I detected a slight smile behind her eyes, which during the days of mask wearing, I had become more observant at seeing. My own smile was hiding behind my mask as well.

Off to the left, a room initially designed for relaxing and connection; it had a large tan sofa, TV, and ample space for sharing a snack on a low table. Eclipsing the ease of gathering, priority seemed to have been given to the books and papers drowning the room currently.

Beth gestured to the woman sitting maskless among the throw pillows, a headset taking her attention and a quick wave to acknowledge my presence without getting up to greet me. I didn't try to wind my way over to reach her either—the stuff surrounding her was a barrier to interactions that day and to painful memories. Her mother, I would soon learn, had filled up Beth's home after her dad had passed away. And although Beth wanted to move forward, to find their floor and their peace again, the greatest obstacle would not be the volume of stuff; it would be her mother's resistance.

Hired at first to help with just one room, the transformation for this family would take much greater effort than a few hours of culling. Deep discussions between a mother and daughter and their therapists would help them move forward, while our organizing efforts could help ensure they would not stay trapped under the wreckage while fighting to get free. For Beth to transform her space she would need to consider the relationships and underlying issues that were all around her at home.

Where we live shapes our lives. In a book about decluttering, we will, of course, discuss what is going on in our homes, and having started with a broader understanding of health concerns related to clutter will help us here also. Building off of the creativity and self-interrogation in the previous chapter, channel that energy into this discussion on the home—because we'll need to be expansive in our thinking to really dissect why the underlying issues that cause clutter in homes comes not just from the stuff lying around us but also our relationships to people, money, and time.

Underlying Issues

Most people pick up a book about decluttering interested in what to do with their homes, so you might be thinking we've finally come to that point after going through all sorts of health challenges first. And yes, we'll talk about such things now, but like in the health chapter, I can't just leave it there. I think the connection between clutter and our homes goes much deeper than your sweater drawer and affinity for large plastic bins.

Recently one of my clients was preparing to move across the United States to start the next phase of his life after getting divorced. He was ready to "rip off all of the Band-Aids" but felt stuck between the excitement the move would offer in terms of freedom and a fresh start, and the familiarity of the items that had been propping up his home and marriage for so long. Discussing what was important to bring with him, and what he was ready to declutter, we had to discern so much about what type life he wanted to establish next: What sort of home would he live in? What activities did he want to do there? Who would be in his life?

Basing his decluttering process around these discussions, a framework emerged for how he could mindfully plan out what was important to consider in terms of home for him. We'll use this framework together in this chapter as the categories offer us a way to work through many of the underlying issues that can present as or relate to clutter in a home. Here are a few examples you'll see throughout this chapter:

1. The Home

- structure
- flow
- beauty (or art)

2. The Stuff

- goals
- clothing
- data-driven organizing

3. The People

- relatives (parents and kids)
- romance (dating, marriage, and partnerships)
- loss

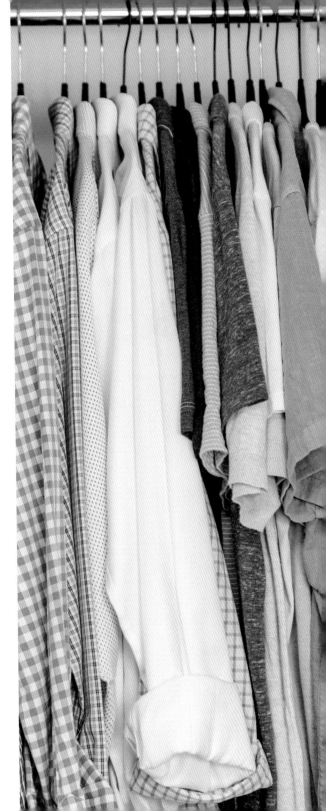

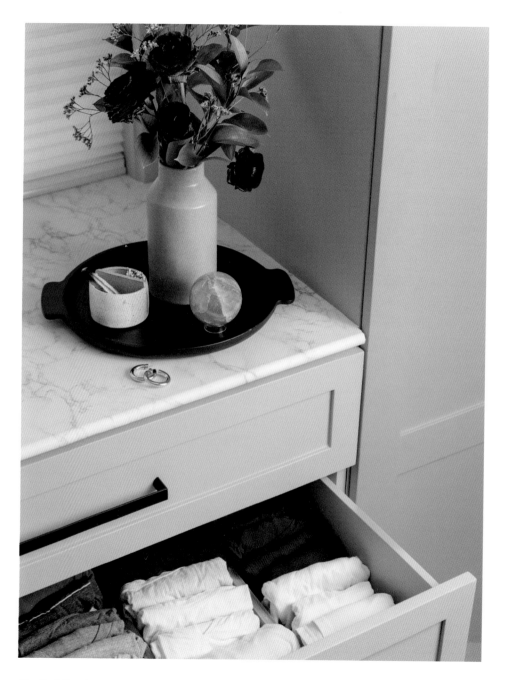

The Home

We introduced the concept of the built environment earlier, and here we'll expand on that. Home-renovation shows have opened people's eyes to how different materials, design choices, and layouts can affect how one lives. When the elements of these categories are put together harmoniously, people can live their lives with ease and have a simple relationship with clutter. When the elements are misaligned with our goals and how we live our lives, chaos and clutter complications have more room to interrupt our plans.

Structure

According to the US Department of Housing and Urban Development (HUD), there are eight principles for a healthy home, which enables "safe, decent, and sanitary housing as a means for preventing disease and injury." The eight principles include:

1. Keep it dry. Prevent water from entering your home through leaks in the roof or poor drainage. Check your interior plumbing for any leaking.

2. Keep it clean. Control the source of dust and contaminants by creating smooth and cleanable surfaces, reducing clutter, and using effective wet-cleaning methods.

3. Keep it safe. Store poisons out of children's reach and make sure they are properly labelled. Secure loose rugs and keep children's play areas free from hard or sharp surfaces. Install smoke and carbon monoxide detectors and keep fire extinguishers on hand.

4. Keep it well-ventilated. Ventilate bathrooms and kitchens and use whole house ventilation for supplying fresh air to reduce the concentration of contaminants in the home.

5. Keep it pest free. All pests look for food, water, and shelter. Seal cracks and openings throughout the home and store food in pest-resistant containers. If needed, use sticky traps and baits in closed containers, along with the least toxic pesticides, such as boric acid powder.

6. Keep it contaminant free. Reduce lead-related hazards in pre-1978 homes by fixing deteriorated paint and keeping floors and window areas clean using a wet-cleaning approach.

Test your home for radon, a naturally occurring dangerous gas that enters homes through soil, crawl spaces, and foundation cracks. Install a radon removal system if you detect levels above the EPA action level. Types of paint, surfaces, cleaning products, and more should be examined.

7. Keep your home maintained. Inspect, clean, and repair your home routinely. Take care of minor repairs and problems before they become large repairs and problems.

8. Keep your home thermally controlled. Houses that do not maintain adequate temperatures may place the safety of residents at increased risk from exposure to extreme cold or heat.

Health at home starts with a framework of good materials and layout you so that you feel well enough to manage clutter. Problems in any of the above categories can lead to health and injury, which can result in serious complications for well-being. But even more unseen structural issues in a home can impact your well-being, particularly clutter. Living in structurally unsafe situations uses up emotional and financial resources which makes it harder to have those resources available for general living.

For instance, access to sunlight helps to regulate mood, energy, and circadian rhythms. When our mood, energy, or our circadian rhythm are out of alignment such as living in a place with no access to sunlight, our executive function will be affected. Having a well-regulated mood and executive function allows us to manage clutter more easily. In the next chapter we will do an exercise focused on this topic.

Flow

The layout of a home is a structural condition, one closely tied to flow or how we move through a space. During home visits with clients, we talk a lot about how they use their space, what areas frustrate them, what they would like to be doing, and how they would like to feel. Then, when we are making decisions about which objects to keep and how to arrange them, we reflect on the activities they plan to be doing there. For instance, if they want an unused room in the house to be a haven for self-care and creativity—rather than be storage for additional stuff—then we decide what to keep based on whether those items align with self-care activities and creativity. This might mean keeping the set of paints and recycling the boxes of paper files that they no longer need. Or, if someone wants a space encouraging their desire to exercise, then we might design that space so there is the preferred exercise clothing and equipment are stored nearby. Closets and shelving that are too high for people to use, making storing items difficult and frustrating, or when the depth of drawers challenges people who are mobility or sight challenged are additional things to consider. This way we are centering choices and values on how they do and will flow within the home. This type of assessment for organizing is a form of human-centered design, which focuses on asking and exploring people's needs and goals (being able to create or exercise at home), rather than starting with a target behavior (decluttering).

The terms surrounding human-centered design have grown in popularity over the last twenty years or so as a description of problem-solving that takes the human perspective into all steps of the process. I heard about this first through program design projects I worked on with the US Agency for International Development (USAID) in connection to work done at Stanford's D School and the organization IDEO. These types of classes and organizations always seemed like amazing places and ideas to me—bringing together humanity's problems and using design to plot a solution. The idea that jobs and trainings like this existed when I was at school in the '90s was unheard of—but it made so much sense to my brain! I took training on these concepts starting around 2014. Later, when I started working as a KonMari consultant, I infused human-centered design into early discussions with my clients to explore how we could set up their homes to suit their lives better, always with their needs and desires at the core of what we did. Let me give you an example of how this approach worked wonders: For my client Rob, we moved all of his exercise equipment to the area of his living room where he would work out so it was convenient. We lowered the height of the shelves in his closet so he could easily put things away as opposed to tossing them up there unsorted. We implemented simple solutions that hadn't been tried before in his home, because he hadn't mindfully taken the time to plan through how he would like to flow in his home or what was helping or hindering what he wanted to do there (like put things away).

This training in human-centered design helped me find greater reasoning behind my work as an organizer. Although it drives some people, I didn't come to this profession just to tidy up shelves so they look pretty—although I do love that beautiful spaces bring some people joy. I enjoy looking for the reasoning behind the decision making, and then transferring that knowledge and the investigatory skills to my clients so they are empowered to continue this type of inquiry and problem solving after I leave them. I help people declutter their lives so that they don't have to spend extra time looking for things or extra money buying duplicates of things they couldn't find. I help people declutter so they can use that time and money to participate in their communities, which in turn can enhance their self-worth, sense of belonging, and positivity.

Home Assessment for Clutter

Time Needed: 15 minutes

Materials Needed: paper, pen, a place to write

Prompt: Read the following passage and write down what comes to mind without censoring yourself.

Pick an ordinary day in your home. Do not clean up ahead of time or nag anyone else to do so. Try to pick your "end of the week" moment—that moment in time when the laundry basket is full, the dishwasher has not yet been emptied, and the stack of mail is about to topple over. Bring your most centered self to this moment. In this reflection, you will be assessing your home like an outsider, so whatever it takes to get to a centered state is important. Perhaps that means a cup of tea or a five-minute meditation or a brisk walk outside. Appreciate that you will be embarking on a new way to consider your space and give yourself an internal cheer to commemorate this time.

First, notice and make a list of the areas in your home. Your areas may include a basement, attic, kitchen, bedroom(s), bathroom(s), workspace (an office or area where work is done), leisure space (designate whether this is shared like a family room or individual like a personal meditation zone), specialized rooms (children's playrooms, laundry room, patio), garage, and pass-throughs (an entryway/mudroom). Now evaluate each area on a scale of 1 to 10 based on how overwhelming the room is. One means "I love this space, and it creates a sense of calm internally." Ten means "if I even look at this space, my face gets flushed, and my temper rises."

Now let's assess the variety and volume of what lives in these spaces. How many types of things does your brain need to register and manage in each of these areas? Does it feel easy to do this or does something stand out that raises your blood pressure? For instance, if the entry area is where you have a lot of shoes, but you also have shoes upstairs in the bedrooms—and also in a box in the attic—take notice of that.

How do you move in these spaces? With ease? With struggle? Let's identify and write down any important structural and behavioral components. "I am in a wheelchair and cannot easily access upper cabinets, so things that live there are useless to me unless my partner gets them" is a structural component related to mobility. A behavioral component might be: "All of the bedroom storage I have is drawers and I hate folding clothes, so my clothes never get folded and end up on the floor."

This assessment of your home is not an indictment of anything; it is a data-generating tool to tease out feelings you have around your things and clutter. It may feel overwhelming at times, but when that happens, take a moment. Take a deep breath. Remember to direct your energy toward the spaces and categories of stuff, which are there to provide you with information. This moment is not for the doing; it is for the noticing. Go throughout your whole living space with this mindset and commit to recording what you see and feel.

Do you live with any other adults or children old enough to participate in this exercise? Involve them as well. Then bring your assessments together to discuss not only what you wrote down but how you felt doing this exercise.

Some specific questions you can consider asking for reflection:

- How do I feel in my home?
- What area do I enjoy being in the most? Why?
- Which objects do I enjoy?
- Are there any zones of tension in my home?
- What bothers me about those areas?
- What do I wish I could do that feels hard to do now?

Use these scores and notes when thinking about where and how to direct your decluttering-related energy and efforts moving forward.

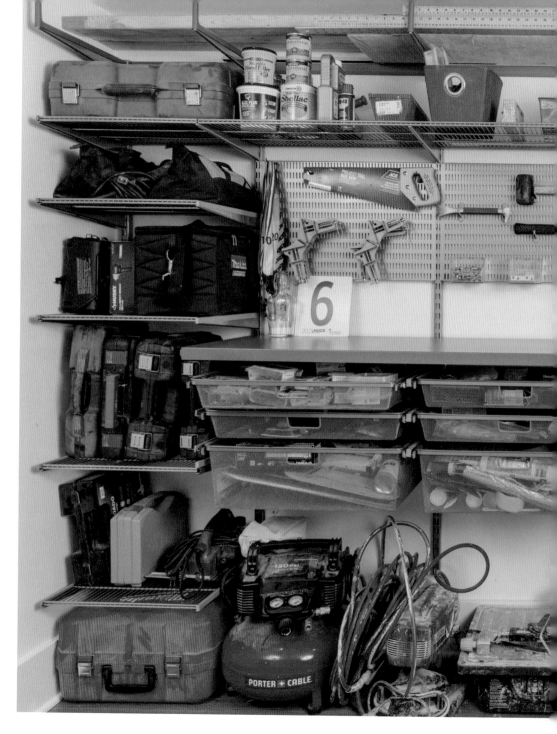

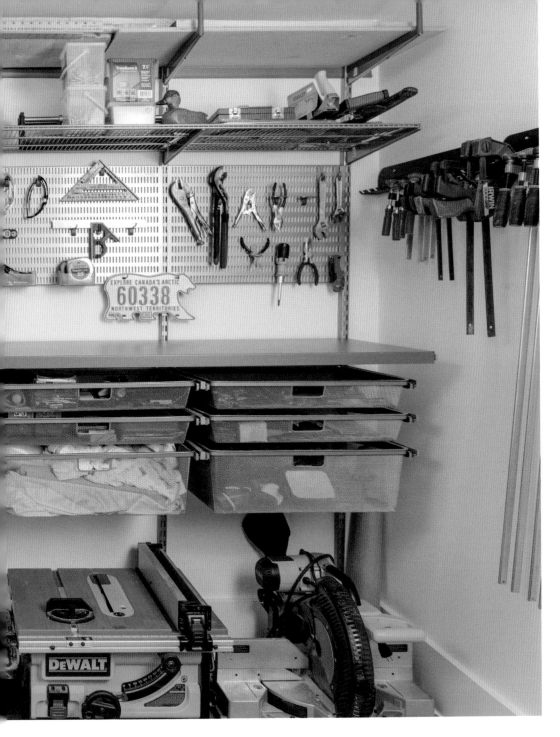

Beauty (or Art)

Clutter can manifest not just as piles of things but as an absence of beauty or art. The buildup of to-do lists and cast offs is draining and uninspiring for the people whose homes I visit. Coincidentally people who suffer with clutter in their homes often put off the enjoyment of bringing art (or of making it visible and enjoyable) into their homes and lives because they feel a disconnect between the beauty of the art and how they feel in their environments. Art is a tool that can help us strengthen our connections to others, to ourselves, and to our environments. If beauty is art and positivity, the absence of such appears as clutter, confusion, and concern.

Please do not confuse my association here as being anti-maximalism, which is a design expression, one driven by the choice to have a high volume of items around. Maximalists often place a premium on surrounding themselves with objects they find beautiful, which can be wonderful when that is their choice, and they can create their ideal environments. This is not hoarding behavior, because that type of accumulation does not come inherently from a place of enjoyment. The differences lie in the intention behind why and how the items we bring into our homes arrive and what emotions they stir inside of us.

I bring this up here to infuse some of the facets of neuroaesthetics into this discussion. The neuroaesthetics field explores the impact of art on the human brain and behavior. Art includes paintings, music, architecture, and any manner of objects and activities. How the brain reacts to external stimuli is key to research in this field, especially the process of perception. Whether we are creating or viewing (or just existing in a room with) art, our brains will release chemicals like serotonin, dopamine, and oxytocin, which induce positive reactions and feelings. This neurological link between what we view or do and how we feel is important.

In the neuroaesthetics field researchers consider both how people experience art as a viewer, listener, or inhabitant (like in a space architecturally), and as a maker of the art in question. Art and design can help frame how spaces are constructed and organized to allow transformations to happen. The experience of living in a home that cultivates experiences that activate your senses positively—a favorite print on the wall, music playing during the day, scented candles lit in rooms—will improve your mood and thus your functioning in that space.

There are some incredible organizations that practice cultivating environments that will foster feelings of well-being and positivity explicitly with their clients. The Oasis Alliance based in the

Washington, DC, area creates sanctuary spaces for survivors of abuse to help them heal. By codesigning personalized spaces for members of the community, the team behind the Oasis Alliance turns homes into places where these survivors can regain their self-worth, heal, and live among beauty and confront their traumatic pasts. Having homes where people feel safe, nurtured, and abundant allows us to experience greater societal goods.

When engaged with the decluttering and design process, art is always on my mind. I like applying the science of the brain to the study of art, and with clients, this means focusing on the art (or lack of) surrounding them. It brings me back to a period when I was depressed in high school and had an urge to paint clouds on the walls of my bedroom. Thankfully this was OK with my parents, and I dotted fluffy white clouds across the light blue walls. The painting process was soothing and then the enjoyment of resting in my room surrounded by these clouds was palpable. Research in neuroaesthetics shows that through certain techniques the brain lights up at the sight of art. Viewing flowers, for instance, may promote feelings of calm. The design of spaces around us can promote or detract from the sense and experiences we wish to cultivate.

So how can we understand what will make our brains light up and then translate those teachings into the design of our homes—and our habits—and keep them? With my organizing clients, I'm always asking questions and listening to pull the thread on how we can use their connections to something from the arts to support their journeys. Temple Grandin reports on one category of neurodiverse people who are visual thinkers, which means they think in pictures. For these people it is likely even more vital to consider art and graphic representation of goals and items in a home when managing clutter. Decluttering with an eye toward cultivating beauty that will make our brains feel positive and calm is a powerful part of the transformation people can experience.

I'd like to introduce some exercises in this book that can bring beauty and art into our lives in small ways. If you feel inspired to expand on these, feel free to do so, and if you feel more comfortable just writing down your answers, that is also OK. But come back to this again someday and try to increase your window of tolerance for this type of activity to see how your experience with your space changes when you incorporate creative activities. Mindfulness practices using different parts of our brains can help us strengthen our connections to our homes through art, and this is one step to take on that path.

Environmental Mapping of the Home

Time Needed: 1 hour initially to take photos and write notes and then add on more time to format the map when you can.

Materials Needed: cell phone with camera; access to any type of document program (e.g., Word or Canva) or pens and paper; a place to write

Prompt: Have you ever mapped your home? This is a great way to evaluate what you have, set boundaries for how much volume you keep of any item, and make it easy to find and put things away. This takes what we have learned in our home assessments and starts to turn it into a system for a decluttered house.

This is especially important for homes where more than one person lives or works—multiple adults who buy things or take grocery trips; children who are always looking for something; and so on. It can serve as a guardrail and reminder about decisions and agreements you have come to about what is important to keep in your home.

For each room or area, take a picture of where things live. For a kitchen, this could include a shot of your pantry, each drawer, and each cabinet. Major spaces that are often included in this type of map include: kitchen, bathroom, sleeping zones / bedrooms, lounging / rest /play areas, and storage zones (basements, attics, hallway closets, etc.). Also, don't be afraid to just draw the spaces, if that is easier for you—

it's your map, so make it look however you want.

If you are taking photos, upload them into a platform where you can add text as well (some examples are a shared Google document or a platform like Notion or Canva). If you are drawing these images, you may wish to have them all collected in a notebook collected or just stored together in a folder on individual pieces of paper.

On top of, or next to, each photo, write the name of what goes there. For a photo of a closet, you may add labels on your image, like "long-hang dresses," "short-sleeved tops," etc. Think in categories here, as broad or specific as makes sense for your life and your things.

For each room or area in your home, write down your answers to the following questions:

- What do I notice about the structure in this space? Are there any concerns about the layout, materials, or lighting I see?

- How do I use and move in this room? Is there anything I wish I could do here that I have trouble doing now?

- What experience of beauty or art do I have in this space? What would I like to add or subtract to make this experience more meaningful?

Once you have all your images and notes put together, it should look like a treasure map, the story of your space, that anyone could pick up and understand where things live in your home and how you feel about them.

As you decide how best to design your Environment Map, think about how you will use it and where it will live. Once you are done, can this live in your digital world, like on Google Drive? Or should it be printed out? It's up to you, but at first, having a hard copy available serves like a training manual with others in your home and in that way is super helpful. This will make it easier to walk around with the manual and talk about it with other people to gain consensus that you are all in agreement that this is where you have decided things should go. Don't be afraid to make more than one version if your discussions prompt changes to where things live or why.

This type of visual map can be especially useful for people with neurodiversity and memory challenges or for parents teaching children how to manage their things. It's also helpful for people who need to have assistance protocols in place. A map helps eliminate the anxiety about not knowing where something is supposed to go, which reduces decision fatigue. And having the underlying reasons clear for the choices made can reinforce the map's validity in mindfully organizing your home.

This can also be a fun activity to get kids involved by having them draw out maps for the items they use most often (toys, books, school supplies, etc.). Being involved in the decision-making about what goes where (perhaps within parameters gently set by an adult) can encourage them to take ownership over putting things away.

Pull out your Environment Map any time someone asks where things go or where something is located. Before embarking on a new hobby or a purchase of a large item, consider the blank space within your Environment Map to figure out if you have room for it.

The Stuff

After going through the Environment Mapping exercise, you will likely be even more aware of the stuff you have and what you are considering to be clutter. Remember clutter can be viewed in simple terms like items that take up space and are either not needed or unorganized. What isn't simple is how it affects us—physically, mentally, emotionally, and even spiritually. When moving from awareness to action it is helpful to keep our overall goals in mind.

Goals

Goal setting can help determine how much decluttering is right for your life, and what its focus can be. It gives us motivation toward a desired result, which makes it easier to flush out the steps we want to take to get there. There are many ways to set goals around decluttering in our homes, and I like to start by figuring out how we can frame them around the reduction of stress.

When I think of clutter causing stress, I remember a client who would always put off addressing her clothing—even after several months of working together. Something else urgent always needed addressed, usually a smaller category or zone in her home, like kids' backpacks and shoes in a clunky corner. That was OK; she was nervous about diving into clothes after several years of changes in her body. She was also exhausted from medical- and life-related challenges, so I had no reason to push her. She naturally brought it up on her own when flights to vacation were coming up. "Maybe next time we could do some of my summer clothes?" she would ask timidly while glancing at the room we had avoided for months. My eyes twinkled with success as I nodded.

And on the day in question, she flowed around the closet—stacks of jeans, which had been feared, were sorted and bagged without tears. We culled shirts and dresses so that there was room to grab a hanger without losing a nail in the search. Stealthily I moved the discard bags to the hallway so her decision-making flow wouldn't be interrupted until at last she looked up and announced, "This is so much less scary than I thought it would be since I practiced with everything else first." Her goal had been to have a closet filled only with items she could, and

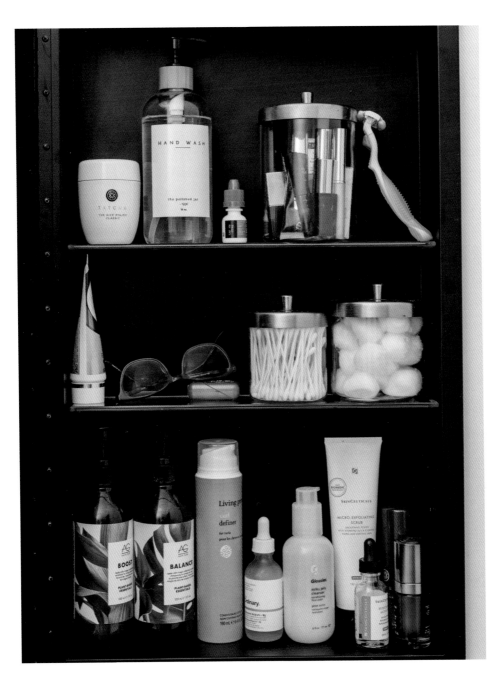

wanted to, wear, and after time spent with my coaching, she had internalized enough of the lessons and their impact on her life to address the area that had first caused her stress.

Goals are important, and how they are achieved may be no less complicated than developing and upholding a mission statement for an organization. The fate of a family may rest on whether the adults are upholding their ends of the agreements they make around distribution of labor and resource allocation and whether or not the children (typically just followers of what the parents deem appropriate until they reach certain ages) are complying with the rules set forth. For adults who live on their own, their household mission statement may be managed by them alone, but it is connected to the external world, their places of employment, their communities, and their broader families and friends. This is because the expectations of society and the environments around us affect how we feel, what we do, and how we spend our resources.

Critically important for goal setting and achievement is this: we need to want to change for ourselves, not for external validation. I see this manifest in the intersection of home and health conditions all the time, such as when a husband hires me to help his wife in her overflowing closet while she is struggling to address the underlying issues of her shopping habit. We may declutter a few bags full of clothes out of the house that day, but likely that is where the movement will end because her goals were not addressed. This makes our session just a Band-Aid that day. Another example is when grant recipients go along with the plans for a health intervention that their donors designed even though they know it doesn't align with the values of the people where it is being rolled out. Misaligned goals and resources lead to tension because they are not motivated from the same source.

When considering how to describe our goals, we need to know what motivates us. Controlled motivation is when our motivation is drawn from gaining rewards or approval or avoiding feelings of punishment and guilt; it is an external form of motivation. For instance, if you feel like you have to work long hours at the office in order to win the approval of your colleagues, this is controlled motivation at work—and it has its pros and cons. Controlled motivation is different than autonomous motivation, when we are motivated by our own psychological needs or internal, intrinsic goals. Maybe you want to work long hours because you really love the project you are working on and relish spending time on it (intrinsic motivation), which is different than staying late to eat dinner at the office because there is a perceived external perception that this is how people show they are committed to the company.

Is intrinsic motivation better than external motivation? Yes, for the long term, absolutely. But in the meantime, experiencing any relief of finishing something can feel amazing. And it can help catapult people toward having their own intrinsic motivation for something they had previously resisted. Getting over the threshold of resistance with some support and being able to move to the next step of the project, or toward your goal, is great. It's also OK to sit with the "I didn't do everything exactly how I hoped to, but it still came out pretty well and I got it done. Phew." That pause in a moment of acceptance and completion can feel pretty good if you let yourself feel it. Often people may start off a new habit—like putting away laundry after it comes out of the dryer—for an external reason (your home organizer suggested to), and over time it starts to feel easier and you start to like the result, so you have internalized the motivation to keep going.

To work toward this shift, it can help to set guardrails (barriers or rules) or arbitrary deadlines along the way. Decision fatigue is exhausting, and sometimes deadlines or self-imposed rules can help us set aside some of that angst. Personally, I have never finished a project without a deadline. My husband has never completed all the items on our house to-do list during a renovation faster than when we had a looming home assessment. Clients who I see regularly will often tell me that they did their homework the morning before I arrived. That's fine! As long as they do it so they can have the experience of feeling that moment and start to spark new neural pathways and then we can continue with the next steps. These small repetitive habit changes over time lead to greater tolerance for a previously challenging task you are trying to routinize on the way toward meeting your goals.

Some things to consider when setting yourself deadlines or guardrails around decluttering:

- Do you have a personal or intrinsic goal related to your clutter?
- Can you define the next steps needed to meet these goals?
- How would you feel if you did not meet your goals?
- What motivation could help you reach your goals?

To declutter your home, we must take time to understand what setbacks you're experiencing. Where do you long to see change? I help people visualize their dream spaces and consider their unique setbacks; only then can we begin decluttering slowly, one next best step after another. And then we can organize and cultivate beauty to reach their visions, until one day my clients are writing me to say that they're sitting in a room they used to avoid, feeling at peace in their homes, and balanced in their daily lives. Those are magical moments.

To get there, let's start with an assessment of our homes as though we were cataloging details to use in a story that can't wait to be told. What do we have? What are the good elements? What are the ones stressing this home system?

Clothing

Has a suit ever brought you to tears? The first time I remember crying in a woman's closet was with a client who worked at the Pentagon. Let's call her "Sally."

Sally was deciding not which clothes sparked joy for her but which ones felt safe—those that let her hide from the gaze of working within a hypermasculine setting. At the Pentagon, she felt a need to cover her curves under baggy suit jackets and slacks because that is the uniform of "the man," which is simultaneously the only outfit that has been deemed "professional" for many environments—even though it was entirely built around a man's body type and traditional fashion sense. Clouding her sense of style and personal emotions and talking about how unfair it all was—and yet how she still needed to have clothes to wear to work—we both cried.

When I moved from Swaziland to DC in 2011, I didn't know what to wear. I'd literally worn through most of my clothes that had been in my closets in Africa for the seven plus years I had lived there, and any still in decent shape as I was getting ready to move, I offered to women I knew before I packed my bags. A DC-based friend told me about a certain style blogger who gave suggestions for women our age working in the stuffy office culture of the city. I started following her and buying the sorts of clothes I thought I was supposed to wear at my job as a Senior HIV/AIDS Advisor at USAID. My favorite outfits for work were my M.M.La Fleur dresses. They made me feel beautiful and smart. A good mix of covered up yet stylish, and I wore wedge heels so I could quickly get down hallways and still feel like I had a bit of height. The M.M.LaFleur dress cuts were not tight, but they did not hide my shape either—I have ample hips, a decent butt, and my Italian grandmother's busty front. I like things that are not too tight around my wrists or hands; to this day if I wear a watch, bracelet, or rings to work, I will take them off when sitting down at a desk. And anything tight around my neck is a no go!

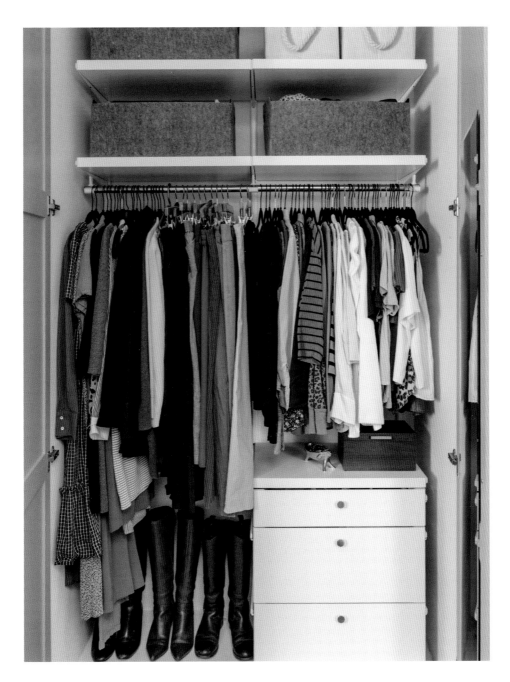

I must have been strangled in a previous life because I hate having tight things around my neck. I also like to be able to slip my shoes off if I am working from a desk. Basically, during those office years, I'd get to work, remove all of my accessories, and tuck one leg under my butt while staring at two monitors. Please message me if you have a credible analysis of this behavior.

Now I have outfits for the two types of work I mainly do—Jenny working at home (computer-based projects) and Jenny working at someone else's home. If you're wondering what I did with all those M.M.LaFleur dresses, I still have two that I wear for events, and the others I eventually sold and donated. For outfits I wear to someone else's home, I have key pieces that allow me to move easily since I do a lot of standing, lifting, and carrying; I also do a lot of sitting-on-the-floor, processing-paper-and-pictures with clients, so I need to be comfortable. My M.M. La Fleur dresses were lovely but would not be ideal for this. I like clothing that does not show my cleavage but is also not a shapeless sack. And I like supportive shoes because I am in my forties and have a bad back. When working at home, I wear a pair of "inside shoes," casual sneakers that I only wear inside so that they do not track in gross stuff. I wear a bra because that kind of support feels good to me, and my hair is pulled up and off my face. It's such a specific and stark difference from how I have existed in other settings.

Feeling very comfortable in my selection of pieces for how I spend my time makes it simpler for me to consider what I need and want to keep around me. I decided to use clothing here as an emblem to carry the discussion on tangible things because of its ubiquity. Pause to think about how the clothing in your life—your patterns of what and how you wear it, your cycles of consumption—are dictated by the external expectations of your world and how that impacts the volume of what you keep around you. This is an internal analysis that can be done whenever you feel identity changes, shifts in regular activities or hobbies or environmental changes.

Data-Driven Organizing

After the goal setting and deciding—oh all of the deciding!—it can finally be time to right size your storage containers based on the final volume of items kept. The internet has lots of visuals and products available to create an organized space. Online searches and external input can work for some people looking to buy products, but usually I just start by using the items my clients already have at home, small boxes from phones or shoes—containers that served a purpose once upon a time—which can all be used when testing out what type of container is best used where. Don't get too hung up with whether or not you have the exact right color or types of containers at this point; those decisions can come over time as you refine your choices and set aside resources to buy new pieces, if that is what you want and need.

Set limits for how much you can buy based on what volume you want to have in your house. You'll have considered some of this already with your environmental mapping exercise. Do you have an extra "just in case" freezer you love to keep stocked? We can get into what food scarcity means for you another time, but I encourage clients to eat through some of the back stock before replenishing items. This also helps reduce food waste since food can expire, go bad, or become no longer something you would like to replenish and consume again. When it comes to clothing, try keeping items one layer deep—one row or drawer of sweaters where you can see everything or one drawer of tee shirts. You get the idea. These are some suggested guardrails that you can modify based on your preferences, access to laundry etc.

What are the measurements that matter in your home? Are there any data points you noticed doing these exercises in your home? In a public health setting, analyzing data points might look like examining a local health center where we see 250 patients queue every day, with a staff of eight nurses and two doctors. This means they each have approximately fifteen minutes per patient. We can extrapolate that they are at a deficit for patient-to-provider ratios, or we know the volume of need is too high for that clinic.

Let's compare that to what is happening in your home. Maybe there are four people who need three meals and two snacks per day, each wear three outfits, which need to be changed each day. This equates to three loads of laundry per week and $800 worth of groceries (do your own math here please!). I recommend you make a list of the activities you get dressed for—office, gym, date nights, etc—and think about how many times per week or month you need those things, divided by how many times you do (or want to do) laundry. Do you have the right amount for what you do? In this type of measurement, we need to prioritize time as the resource to manage feelings of being overwhelmed since everyone's budget and financial situation will be vastly different. If we want to change our time allocations, do we redistribute the load (have more people spend fewer hours each per week doing laundry) or are there tasks we can shift so that different people do different things?

Volume is one of the categories that can cause the most tension in a home. Developing a set number of things before ordering more (i.e., only five swimsuits at a time) is important.

Remember that guardrails, like limits, are meant to help us reach our decluttering goals: they are not meant to be punitive. That said, sometimes people rebel against limits. If you'd like to try to get yourself out of the habit of over buying, consider this example I used with a client who was constantly buying more clothing than her grandson needed: whenever you find yourself about to purchase something you already have enough of, look at the dollar amount of what you were supposed to spend. Take that amount and add it to a note you keep on your phone called "charity donations." Over time that note should probably start looking like "$14, $32, $27." The pause between buying the item you saw and writing down the amount on your list is about widening your window of tolerance so you can sit for a moment and think about why you are about to make a purchase and whether it is necessary. You may still decide to purchase the item but keep writing down the dollar amounts anyway. Set yourself a monthly reminder to look at the total listed on the charity donations note and then donate that amount to a cause that matters to you.

The pause between stimulus and response encourages you to take stock of what you are doing and make a more conscious decision about where to put your resources. Mindful organizing in action. Over time, check out the bigger change you've helped make happen by reallocating your consumption habits toward charities you support. That client, who changed her habit, later expressed to me that she felt vulnerable at first when encouraged to look so closely at her spending—it is important to note that I did not ask to see this note or how much she was spending; that would be a surefire way to increase her shame. But when she made her first donation after a few weeks of tracking the "almost purchases," she felt some relief. This made it easier for her the next month to continue with the habit and slowly reduce the times she purchased clothes for her grandson, which was her original goal.

Someday/Maybe

In our home, we need systems in place to track our habits—especially our spending habits, since most of us live in a consumerist society with advertisements all around us. That's why I often suggest making a someday/maybe list. It's a good cousin to your Ideas Home discussed in the next chapter. This is a list on which you can put all those items that pop up that you typically would have bought right away (a cute sweater on sale, the latest bestseller from your favorite author, etc.). If you've taken the brave step to get a handle on what is living all around you, I'd rather you not sabotage yourself during the process by bringing in more items before you've had the chance to experience what it feels like to live with what you really need and want and use.

I've had a someday/maybe list on my phone in the reminders section since 2011, when I first learned about this concept from a course I took at work taught by Lindsey Satterfield, who was teaching us David Allen's *Getting Things Done* method. I've added or subtracted things over the years. I've used it when my mother asks me what I want for a holiday gift or when I refresh my wardrobe or bookshelves. Putting something on the list generally allows me to get the nag of desire off my mind. But what if it isn't that easy for you? Do you need something a bit stricter? Something that brings in that mindful pause before you make a purchase you don't really need?

Ready to make your list? Try these ideas to get started:

- Establish the list in an easy to access container (notes app on your phone, daily planner, etc.). Start off by adding items that you are waiting to buy right now—a book by your favorite author that hasn't launched for presale yet, or the brand name you prefer for sweaters due to arrive in a few months. During your decluttering process it is especially important to use this list to add items to categories you are decluttering otherwise the never-ending influx of new items will obscure the progress you've made.

- Remove or delink your credit card(s) from any browser that automatically tracks them for shopping. Find yourself on eBay all the time? Remove your credit card info so that you'd have to go fish it out of your wallet across the room before making a purchase. Even better, tape a sticky note on your card that says, "Do I really need to use this now?"

- Reallocate your shopping habits to a cause that matters to you. You could set up a note on your phone and keep track of the money there of money you *almost* spent on "x thing" and instead, donate that accumulated amount at the end of each month. The point is the redirection of the money. The intention is a shift from unchecked consumerism to community assistance.

- Consider asking for something from your "someday/maybe" list from a relative, friend, or partner, when they ask you what you'd like for an upcoming holiday. People often love knowing that they are getting you something you have want but might not purchase for yourself.

Seven Rings aka the Stuff Budget

Time Needed: 30 minutes initially

Materials Needed: paper, pen, a place to write, and the Environment Map you made earlier

Prompt: Does what we buy fit into our homes at a level that does not overwhelm us?

"I see it. I like it. I want it. I got it." With apologies to Ariana Grande, whose song "7 Rings" lives rent free in my head, this behavior will drown your home (and possibly take all your money).

The Environment Maps you made earlier created an objective look at what is living where in your home. Now let's add another layer to look at the spending habits that brought in these items and evaluate how you feel about that through the lens of decluttering.

Look at the zones you wrote about in your Environment Map, category by category and reflect on the volume of each. Does it feel like the right amount? Who purchased or provided the items for this category? How does the volume of what you have meet your goals (or not)?

For any category where the volume you are reviewing feels off, set boundaries on how much of it you wish to have in your home at any given time. Figuring out the right amount of each category you want to have on hand could be an amount

that fits within the space allocated on the map, aligns with your goals, and adjusts to your budget.

Now that you have done this, let's think about the zones throughout your home that might have had more space. If you have storage areas with empty space, you may notice you have the opportunity to bring things in for new activities, or you can point these out to the parents or relatives who send unrequested items over to communicate that you have not allocated space for new things.

As always, this is best done after you have decluttered the different categories of items in your home. I recommend the KonMari Method™ for this part of the work—it is a structured and mindful approach to decision-making, using joy as a metric for what to keep and what to let go of. For more about that, check out Marie Kondo's book, *The Life-Changing Magic of Tidying Up*. It helps guide many of the steps of my work with clients, and I am indebted to her for the impact the book and her method has had on my life.

If you can make that shift toward reallocation, you may experience a growing desire to pause the "auto-buy" part of your brain and make a difference. A small but accumulating difference. With the same client mentioned above, we were already making furniture donations of pieces she no longer needed in her home to a local group—Homes Not Borders (HNB)—who were helping resettle new Afghani refugees into the DC area. I asked her to put their online donation link in her phone in an open browser—most of the shopping she was doing was through her phone—so that every time she looked up some clothing online, she could take that amount and add it into a donation she would make to HNB instead. This is one way that decluttering is not just about "less stuff" as much as it is about increased awareness of how much we consume, where we can upcycle our belongings, and how we can contribute to our global community in a way that is more meaningful.

The People

For a good chunk of my life, I helped lead programs to change sexual behavior or adopt voluntary medical procedures for HIV prevention. When I started my professional-organizing career, I confess that I thought, *Oh, tidying a home will be so much easier!* But no—that was a mistake. Interpersonal dynamics from the bedroom spill into the closets, the kitchen, and the living room, and they affect our everyday well-being profoundly. A disagreement over the spice drawer becomes animosity toward weekend plans. Not having your needs met sexually leads to arguments about closet space.

Most of life happens in the everyday boring moments—putting your clothes away or not, washing dishes, storing keys in a place that makes sense. These everyday moments can impact how we feel since they make up a lot of time in our lives. This means that if we don't deal with the emotions that decluttering brings, interpersonal dynamics can become fraught. In Eve Rodsky's 2019 book *Fair Play: A Game-Changing Solution for When You Have Too Much to Do (and More Life to Live)*, she shares that 25 percent of couples divorce over everyday home discrepancies.

Chaos at home may be familiar to many of us, especially if we grew up around it. This can manifest as a fear of success about decluttering, which may be a deeper fear of moving past where we were growing up and becoming different than our parents—even if we know that something was wrong with our childhood environments. Therapy can help in this healing process, where people are examining who they are, where they come from, and who they want to be. With greater awareness brought about through this type of deep introspective work, making changes in how you approach decluttering compared to what you knew growing up does not have to be riddled with shame. With strong intrinsic goals and practice establishing boundaries it becomes easier to see how your choices today (whether around how many gifts you allow your children to receive or what you want to do with every copy of a magazine that arrives at your house) are not indictments on your parents, but rather choices—just that—that you feel empowered to make and voice.

Brené Brown—patron saint of vulnerability—asks her audience through her work on "living big," what boundaries need to be in place for you to be in your integrity and generous in your assumptions about others? Take a few moments to reflect on what this means for you in the context of your home. Do those boundaries look like setting limits on how many items are allowed to be sent home with you from an aunt after a holiday meal? Do they look like offering one afternoon a month to sit with an aging parent to help sort through photos and old clothes?

Decluttering a home based on your goals and needs can help offset potential tension you may experience with relatives over your decluttering choices when you focus on creating spaces that nurture connection and communication. Priya Parker's book *The Art of Gathering: How We Meet and Why It Matters* offers many suggestions we can use for how to consider decluttering your space with connection in mind, if that is your goal. First, how would you define what types of connection and communication you want? Do you want to have a big dining room table so you can invite people over and share meals easily? Many people say they want to host gatherings but feel ashamed by their clutter, so they don't. Other people feel anxious about the idea of hosting and prefer intimate gatherings or online connections. In that case, consider how you can connect with people virtually (through games, screens, devices, decent Wi-Fi, etc.) and what kind of space would make it enjoyable to do that? For example, if you have kids who can be noisy, you might need a quiet room where you can sit in a comfortable chair and FaceTime with your friend while someone else takes care of the kids during your weekly phone calls. Once you know what types of communication and connection you want, we can move into the dynamics of the people you want there.

My fascination with family dynamics and clutter probably stems from the class that made me want to become a sociology major in college, "Family and Intimate Relationships." When I started college, my parents were going through a traumatic divorce so no wonder that class title appealed to me. I was eighteen and trying to intellectualize what was happening in my own family to see if it would predict my future. It's little wonder my career has progressed into examining how intimate relationships affect whether we do or do not have certain health conditions and how we manage the chronic challenge of clutter. I was initially interested in how intimate relationships related to HIV transmission and how infectious diseases are contracted, but now I examine how family relationships do or do not share the household load and how this contributes to clutter and mental health problems for my clients.

Sex is complicated as a field of study, and it can be in practice too. In my youth, I assumed sex was the most intimate experience people could have but then I discovered joint checking accounts and parenthood. But seriously—I've been in the bedrooms and closets of people all over the world, and I have seen so many parallels between navigating sexual practices and preferences and those of purchasing habits and organization.

After studying sex, I moved into studying the behaviors around sex. My work on behavioral-change campaigns earlier in life included supporting women to practice condom negotiation and request HIV tests. Those same communication and negotiation skills are what people in my DC neighborhoods use to ask their partners to finish putting up those goddamned shelves in the living room so they can finally put away their things.

Communication and negotiation skills are important for behavior change, and also for diplomacy (the art of dealing with people in a sensitive and effective way). Switching from working for the US State Department as a diplomat to working for myself as a professional organizer I've had enough experience to know that these skills are as important when representing your country to heads of state as it is for helping adults who live together manage a conflict over where piles of mail live. Decluttering our homes also deserves this level of sensitivity and efficiency. As a diplomat in Swaziland, I had to negotiate with the king and various government leaders when our US Ambassador brought me along to lots of different offices to pitch our policies and programs. My job was to align our mission with the internal goals of their offices. Minister of labor? Reducing HIV infection rates would help keep more workers alive longer. Transport? Same thing. We were trying to generate demand for service or activities that met correlated goals of these leaders. Our goals intersected around adjusting policies (like allowing workers to have paid time off to get HIV tests) or structural issues (like providing private spaces at work for lactating mothers). Using this same approach can be helpful when dealing with people whose actions affect clutter in their homes. Truly decluttering a space requires more than reorganizing a room; it is about understanding the underlying issue and changing behaviors or structural factors to support the goal being met.

The impact of a cluttered space on our minds and habits overwhelms many people, and we've talked about some of the reasons why this happens—and why it manifests more strongly for some people. Treating the relationship people have with clutter compassionately is so important, especially if you have a goal of a peaceful home. Examples of how clutter manifests in homes include losing things, buying too much of unneeded things, and spending too much time picking up things. These things cause arguments with loved ones, which I notice manifest as resentment over in-laws bringing more stuff or one partner thinking items should stay longer in a space longer than the other wants. Clutter becomes an emotional barrier between what we have and what we want out of life.

Family

From my clients, I hear both sides of stories like, "My mother always told me I was wrong for keeping things" or "My mother cried whenever something was thrown out." I had one client who was always anxious about his wife's organizing sprees because he could only connect them to his mother's hoarding behavior. Because of this he didn't participate in organizing their home, which created tension between them.

What were the lessons you learned about stuff when you were a child? How have they stayed with you in obvious or surprising ways?

As adults, these lessons can make us question what the right choices are to make with our things. But the people who reach out to me—mostly between the age of thirty-five and fifty-five—are adults who know they want to do and live differently in their homes than they are currently, they just might not know how to do so. That desire is vital. Becoming free of the fear of becoming like the stories we remember as children means breaking the consumerism cycle, like always buying things you don't truly need just because they are on sale and breaking the self-sabotaging patterns of financial habits that resulted in the over accumulation of goods.

Talking with Your In-Laws about Gifts

What are the conversations we need to have, or the boundaries we need to put into place with family members, to honor our priorities and to help us meet our clutter-related goals?

Here is a conversation starter for in-laws who send us too many things. By far in every workshop I've ever offered related to decluttering, one of the top questions is always around this topic. The general script can be modified too based on whoever in your life is contributing to excess in your home. Foundationally we want to underscore the connection between you and whoever you are speaking to, sharing facts about your situation more than making accusatory statements, and offer an on ramp (gradual approach) to the desired behavior change. Give this a try:

"Hey, I wanted to let you know what we are doing this season. We are decluttering our home so it can make us feel better! You might know that we've been (insert 'stressed out, spending too much money on purchasing things,' etc.), and we are spending so much time cleaning up that we don't have time to connect and play anymore (insert your goal). We want to change this situation, so we can enjoy our lives together more. To that end, we are going to ask that you take a pause on giving us things for our house or the kids. This doesn't mean forever, but for now this is what will help us feel good."

Going into this conversation, practice ahead of time with a partner or friend. Attach the meaning behind this decision (that you feel stressed) so it takes the pressure off of their actions (sending you too much stuff) and puts it on the items and your desire for improvement in your home life.

When should you do this? As soon as you start decluttering your home or approaching your things more mindfully. Start to sensitize them to the idea of this "influx pause." It might take a few discussions before they agree to it, but just like any change in behavior, slow improvements or repetitive action over time become more meaningful and sustained the longer you practice them. I often suggest that my clients start talking to their parents (or whoever is sending them unnecessary stuff) about our work together since it may help to point out this change in behavior to a neutral party at first.

There are many ways a disconnection in what we want as adults and how we were raised can present or be caused. Epigenetics for instance, is the translation of experiences from our parents to us as unborn children, and how early childhood experiences (e.g., trauma) can lead to destructive behaviors as adults. Abuse and terrible situations at home can lead to complex PTSD and estrangement from family members, which can also result in a disconnection from other communities and the ability to thrive in the world. Feelings of safety and attachment can help people rebalance their lives. Examples of developing safety include healthy relationships, nonscarcity mindsets, healthy buying habits, and therapy. If you have low self-esteem because of guilt and shame related to how you grew up, consider this question: Who would you be if you didn't feel badly about yourself? What type of support would help you realize your desires?

Mindfully processing experiences we have had, and then thoughtfully and carefully changing behavior around these ideas can help you along this process of growth. These changes can help people break the cycle of clutter in their homes and allow people to be happier, which then leads to more fulfilled lives in their homes and beyond. Setting a pattern for your home to address chaos and clutter mindfully and regularly will help support your goals for the future. One next best step after another next best step.

The Impact of Personal Stories

In 2019 I had a long string of work trips to visit women's health clinics across southern Africa to see how effective a cervical cancer program my organization supported was for women in those countries. Those days were filled with long drives, chatty coworkers, and my favorite roadside snack: a chicken meat pie. Everywhere I went, we interviewed female clients who had gone through the programs to get their input—shocking but interviews were not always done during site visits, which were often centered around reviewing data registers. Researchers involved in this work often focused on quantitative measurements of change or success, such as metrics that showed improvement or failure rates of cervical cancer. Numbers and data are helpful, yes, but only when they mean something *to* and *for* the people they are designed to support. As it stood, the numbers around cervical cancer were not effective by themselves in moving people to change their behaviors. I wanted to know how long it took for women to get somewhere they could get a service, what happened when they got there, how they felt, and how they were treated by family members involved in their health care decisions. As their advocate and the person who would take their voices and turn that into policy changes, money, or life improvements, I felt a sense of responsibility to contribute to their well-being. I feel similar with my organizing clients.

It's not enough to run numbers and data by people and expect radical behavior change. The impact of personal stories around the impact of clutter can hopefully help though, one reason I've included so many in this book. I want to go into my clients' offices, talk to their bosses, and explain that if their staff had three hours each week to complete ordering and returns, to make that dentist appointment, or to incorporate fifteen minutes of stretching into their daily schedules, they would feel less overwhelmed. I want to talk to their health insurance providers about why getting help from a KonMari-type organizer would be a perfect complement to the therapy sessions they are receiving to process having grown up with a hoarder—couldn't those sessions be discounted? I want to talk to your husband or wife and explain how certain household changes will help to get the house in shape but that it is not a one-time thing. Rewiring the brain takes repetitive actions over time. You have to keep wearing the condom, putting the toilet paper away in the right place, taking fifteen minutes to meditate every day. I've seen how lasting behavioral, structural, and biomedical changes can decrease a national HIV transmission rate, curb employee burnout, and save families—and I know similar results are possible for decluttering.

Sometimes I feel like I am bearing witness and validating the inner knowledge my clients possess. Like, "Yes, it is OK to throw out the receipts you saved from five years ago," and "No, you do not need to keep the ugly tablecloth your mother-in-law sent you." Where has our inner knowing gone? Why have we been unable to assert ourselves when something feels off? It has made me more conscious of the validation I have sought too. I ask myself questions for further clarification, like, "Am I posting on social media for likes and attention or am I posting because I know that what I have to say matters?" In this case, the behavior of "posting on social media or not" has an intermediary question, where I check in with my "why." I ask my clients to tap into their inner knowing too, which requires a lot of self-reflection and radical honesty. I learned in my interviews with people during my public health career that support structures are vital. For instance, many women needed their health care providers to talk to their husbands and their mothers-in-law to get them on their side so they could go for procedures; this can be done in other areas as well. I often act like a patient advocate for my organizing clients, helping them negotiate chores or time to have their medical visits. I think of this as a form of doula work—caring and guiding someone through all the steps of decreasing feeling overwhelmed, like an HIV case manager or

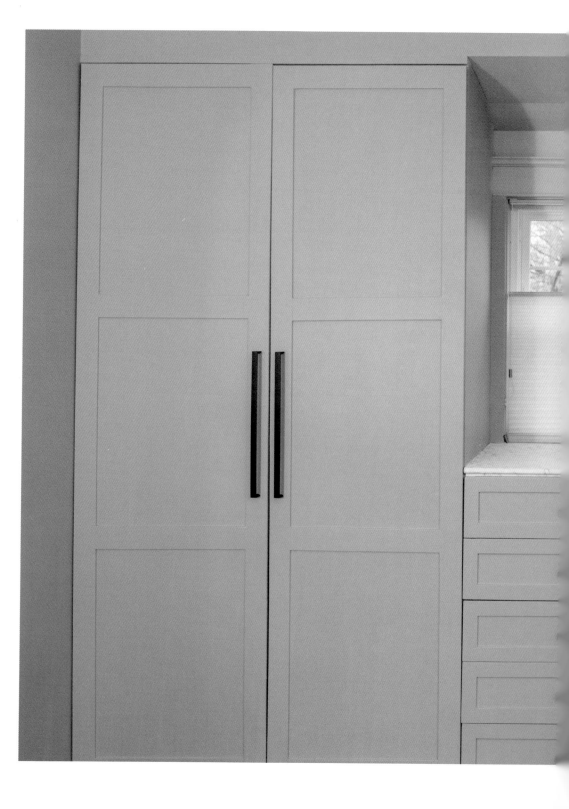

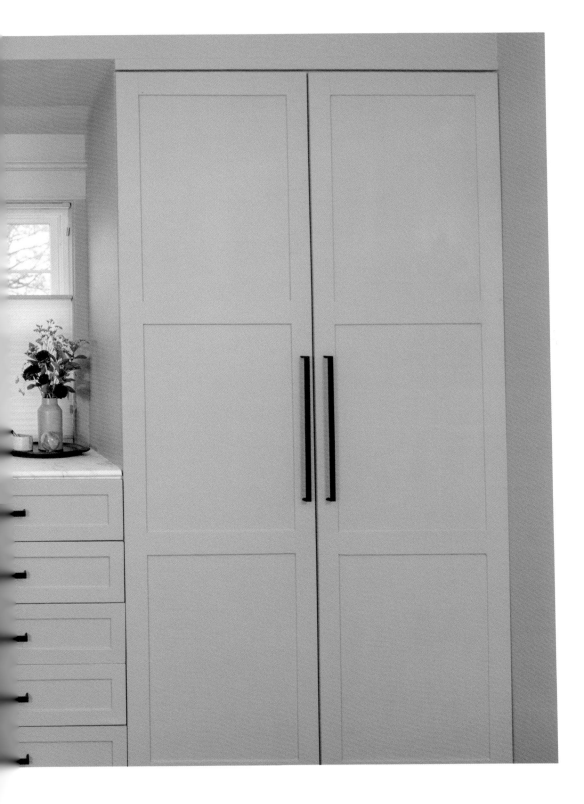

community health worker (CHW). We all need care—community-based care like that discussed in the health chapter, be it strangers or neighbors or family or friends or teachers—for different areas of our lives. Caseworkers and CHWs help guide patients through challenging situations or transitions into new phases in their lives. They are wise and caring (or they are supposed to be) and hopefully neutral unlike family members. Unfortunately, emotional labor is not usually paid well or endorsed by the structures that form our societies, which is why many CHWs are over-worked, burnt out, and exhausted.

I have been in hundreds of homes of stressed-out people. I have worked in offices where stressed-out people caused further harm. I have worked with hospitals where patients had pre-ventable diseases and ailments caused by others. Hurt people hurt people is a common refrain. This happens on an individual level in terms of abuse within families, but it also happens in the broader context of policies that cause harm to others. I started my business in Washington, DC, because I was living there at the time but also because I knew the power that people around me yielded. They were in charge of policies and budgets and programs affecting millions of peo-ple around the world—and I saw their stress all the time. The more I talked about my interest in home organizing, the more people related to how that affected their own lives. People want to be listened to, acknowledged, and supported. At home their concerns are dismissed. At work they are pushed to the side. People even dismiss themselves—how extreme this is depends on how they were raised. *Where can we find feedback and assurances on our life choices grounded in compassion?* We will come back to this question around permission and compassion in the next chapter when we explore decluttering relationships too.

Children

"The mean tidy lady took my toys!" was not a phrase I thought would ever be uttered in my direc-tion, but one Sunday afternoon, in a large, painstakingly renovated home in upper northwest DC it happened. I had been wounded by a seven-year-old who could no longer find the soccer ball her mother had placed in a basket under the stairs because she blamed me for its absence.

I don't have my own children, but for the most part, I like other people's kids.

"Why do you always make a mess with Ms. Jenny?" said a five-year-old who I promise you made *way* bigger messes than I did. That was partially why his mother had hired me: this child's messes, his dad's messes, and her messes were overwhelming all of them. I took a breather before answering this child's question, my hands wrapped around a giant stuffed koalaand said: "Sometimes you need a big mess to realize you need a big change."

Although kid related clutter is often a cause of stress, I recommend applying the same logic and analysis to it that we discussed around clothing earlier. Keeping in mind that children usually have no participation in the accumulation of the items and age-appropriate discussions are recommended for how to help them learn to keep things mindfully organized.

Romantic Relationships

When I moved back to the States in 2011, I was excited about two things: to live near a well-stocked grocery store and to start dating online. Online dating had become a common practice during the seven years I was living overseas, where my lack of a smartphone and intermittent internet access made such an activity impossible. Loosely involved with an unobtainable man I had met at a work event (also the subtitle of my next book) made me all the more excited to pursue all of the options available within a ten-mile radius of downtown DC. (Virginia and Maryland addresses need not apply.) But my transition was hard. One day, I had a meltdown in Whole Foods while staring at the excess and abundance of food in contrast to the Swazi shops I had recently made do at. And the online dating scene made my eyes blink wide and my heart leap in fear. This was not the transition back to America I had imagined.

Online dating in DC, basically my side job on and off for seven years, felt like the 2016 roller coaster election cycles—exciting and promising but ultimately dangerous and full of lies and unfulfilled fantasies. Finally, I met someone in my mid-thirties who seemed reasonable, and we moved in together. Success? Maybe, except he had a drinking problem. This was supposed to be better, he convinced me, because he used to have a drug problem. And because I had never lived with an addict before, I took his word for it. The bottles of whiskey started to pile up. One day I said, "Oh, let's start keeping these and then we can use them to serve water for dinner parties or as vases." These were the years when this was trendy décor at dimly lit restaurants with brick walls. He seemed not to care until the bottles began stacking up and up and up along the wall and the reality sunk in that all the thirsty dinner guests in the world couldn't match whatever pain he was drinking away.

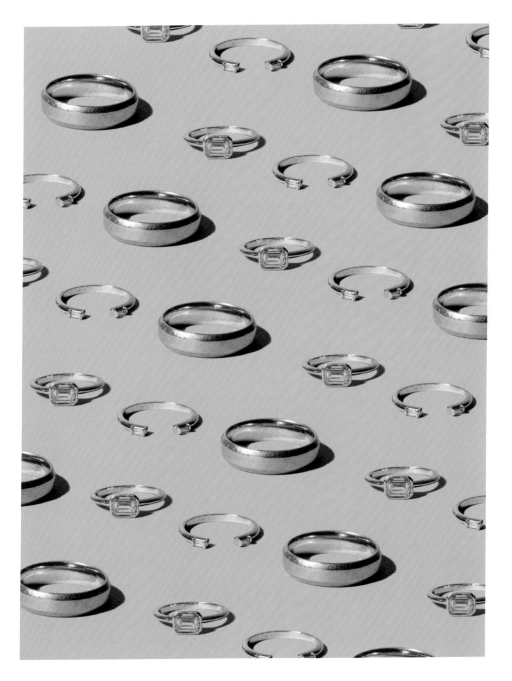

As part of my training for KonMari certification, he participated as one of my practice clients—honestly one of the nicest things he did for me in that season of our lives—and during one moment of reviewing his things together he said, "I don't know if I bring you joy anymore—I don't know if we bring each other joy anymore." It was sad and nothing came of the discussion until months later, on January 1. He woke up in the morning and told me he was leaving. I was devastated at the time—and although it was painful, I now know how vital that was for my growth and future happiness. I know it all stemmed from asking these questions about what joy meant in our lives. Where did our joy go? Where did my joy go?

I recycled all those bottles years ago but looking at collections of glass vases and containers still reminds me of him. That build-up of glass clutter symbolized our problems—his drinking and my not acknowledging the fear I had of being alone. I choose unsafety rather than being alone.

I see now that my feelings of self-worth were tied up in partnership and cluttered my ability to connect with the right kind of partner. My dating mindset at the time was "anything is better than nothing." I couldn't recognize that having less, being single, would have been better for me. The attachment I felt to being needed, wanted, and validated as part of a couple was hard to shake. It required me to look deeply inside and be honest with myself. I'd sunk a tremendous cost (time, emotion) into dating someone who wasn't a good match for me, not unlike the too tight and too bright club clothes of my early twenties.

The shortest uncoupling of clients I have worked with was about twelve minutes. I'd arrived at their house—a boyfriend and girlfriend living together—to begin our decluttering work. The girlfriend had worked with me two years earlier when she lived on her own in a cute apartment with good light downtown. We sat on the couch and chatted about their vision for the session and what we would focus on—but it was quick because we had a phone call the previous week on the same topic. Then we walked through the rooms of the two-story home, focusing on areas of congestion and where we might set up to work on clothing that day for both of them. I was in the living room shaking out some garbage bags to get ready for the donation piles when the couple, whispering in the corner of the kitchen, said they were going to step out to the back porch for a moment to talk. I sat down on the couch. Twiddled my thumbs. Double-checked that my phone was on silent. Let my eyes roam around the room. Ten minutes later the boyfriend walked in and over to the bedroom. He snagged a backpack there, mumbled a quick, "Nice to meet you," to me on his way out the door, and left. The girlfriend, hovering near the kitchen, firing off texts, watched him leave and sighed. "He's leaving," she said. "Oh, OK," I said, "should we get started without him? Will he come back later to join us?"

"No," she said, "he just left, left. Well, technically his name is on the lease, so I will have to leave, but he is gone for the rest of the day. We just broke up."

I know I didn't cause their breakup, but my presence had triggered something for them—committing to decluttering and organizing that day echoed a much more serious commitment assumption, one that they were not prepared to take together.

Other couples have broken up months or years after we started working together. Stress caused by clutter is a good reason for families to try to change the dynamics, if they want to stay together, and sometimes that does work. Relationships change and grow stronger as communication improves, and often—in tandem with therapy—people work through issues together. But also, as the clutter clears, so does the illusion of relationships that have been held together by the piles of crap covering the floors.

I became a type of marriage counselor during my KonMari sessions way before I was actually married. Placed in the middle of couples who had been living together for years and had recently hit a breaking point about who was putting what where, I was helping meditate compromises and practice behavior change so that harmony could ensue in the house. Favorite clients of mine started our work together letting me know they had been married for thirty-five years and wanted to stay that way if I could only help them navigate their downsizing journey.

What I was seeing was that clutter can manifest in a marriage in many different ways, like unequal roles and responsibilities, differing opinions over household management and purchasing, and having too many ideas about how life is supposed to be lived at home. Looking to find shared intrinsic motivation around behavior change I often turned to my old work subject: sex. This was something that often partners are in favor of experiencing together. In a male reproductive health program I had worked on years earlier, we found that men were most motivated to get circumcised when the women they wanted to sleep with said they liked circumcised penises better. Shared motivation at play. So many people feel the same way about a clean countertop—it's hard to feel sexy and close to someone when physical clutter and a mess of decisions are swirling all around you.

This may or may not resonate with you, but perhaps you have your own shared motivation with your romantic partners. What drives you toward shared goals? How can that become linked to solving issues around clutter in your home?

Demand Generation

Generating collective interest in reducing clutter in our homes may need the cooperation of different people in our lives. Demand generation increases awareness of and demand for health products or services among a particular intended audience through social and behavior change communication (SBCC) and social marketing techniques. Trying out different techniques with people you share a relationship with can open new lines of communication and offer opportunities for improvement and to reach your decluttering goals.

Demand generation in relationships is how we inspire people to act in ways that are more aligned with a decluttered mindset for the home. When I was able to communicate with my husband that having a clean apartment helped me relax, which made it easier for me to get in the mood for sex, his demand was generated to keep our home tidy.

If this resonates with you, you may ask: How do I deal with clutter in relationships and prevent it from getting worse? Consider the following exercise like screening questions or a relationship check-in when trying to get on the same page about decluttering with a partner to see where your compatibility is aligned or where it could use some tending. Many people go through assessments of how their skills match up with potential jobs, but rarely do anything as rigorous when evaluating potential partners. This is a shame since our relationships impact so much of our lives, especially within a home.

Loss

Thousands of bells sat silently on shelves in wooden cabinets throughout the house. A mother's never-ending collection had become a stumbling block for the daughter left to empty and sell her parents' home after their unexpected and premature deaths. Her own home, business, and children puttered along as she went back to the house week after week, each time overwhelmed by grief and the volume of items, unable to decide what to do next. Small treasures her mother had accumulated over the years were individually unimportant, but when experienced all together—in their home—they were as momentous as the void created by her death. Her own papers from work on an important legal case stored in the garage were far less important and difficult to deal with than the tiny trinkets throughout her mom's house.

Generating Demand for Decluttering

Time Needed: 20 minutes

Materials Needed: Partner or family member with whom to generate demand

Directions:

Sit together and have a pen and piece of paper each. Take three minutes to write down your thoughts on the following questions. Some of these are similar to earlier questions I suggested for self-reflection, but in this context, we want to consider our shared experiences with someone for whom you hope to generate demand for interest in decluttering your home.

- How do you want to feel in your home?
- What do you want to be able to do there?
- What do you want to see when you walk into the space?

Next, think about the challenges that interfere with decluttering in your home. Write down anything that comes to mind. After you have written your notes, share those feelings with each other. No need to make blaming or judging statements, just let each person speak—without interruptions—for three minutes during the first round of sharing. Focus frustrations on the items or practices that might have come up, rather than the people (for now). Frame your discussion around shared priorities for the home as a way to direct the discussion.

A family home filled with items, often loved, used, and treasured during life, may turn into a space of sadness after the relatives die—compounded in grief by the time and money it takes to deal with the items. It is a quick transition of emotions that can be experienced in spaces like these: one moment filled with love and laughter, the next with loss and responsibility. Some of the responsibilities can be avoided if dealt with earlier, say if elderly parents begin to declutter their things while still active. For many of us though, getting our parents to do anything we want is a challenge: my own mother resisted decluttering her possessions until six and half years after I became a professional organizer, all the while I stewed and calculated the number of weeks it would take me to empty out her home someday. I didn't want her to die but I had an almost anticipatory sense of grief knowing so well that I would have to put aside my grieving for losing her in favor of closing out her estate. For children—even adult children—who are responsible for their family members' things, anticipatory grief can mount as they watch their parents' homes fill to the roof with idiosyncratic collections and rising rebellion against downsizing. We must ask ourselves if our parents' passions will become our pain points.

Like the stages of grief themselves (denial, anger, bargaining, depression, and acceptance) we will flow through similar moments when decluttering after a loss. Having someone with you go through this type of decluttering process can offer a way to talk through the stages, mirror and validate emotions you are feeling, and support you in getting the necessary tasks done.

For instance, if left with boxes and boxes filled with paperwork and photographs after a parents' death there will be mixed emotions going through them. Some of my clients start off angry at this burden and use our sessions to say things that would be discouraged in front of other family members like "How dare they leave me so many boxes in drawers full of paperwork and photos for me to deal with after their death! Why were they so selfish?" But those feelings move along the grief spectrum as we work through the items. I was sorting dozens of tubs worth of photos with one of my clients, labeling each photo by event type, and we saw her parents on cruises in the Caribbean and on European trips that she didn't remember them ever taking. On family holiday after family holiday, their smiles and the fact they had ordered doubles of all the prints showed how much joy they were having in their lives. "Oh, yeah, they loved living life. They did not rest at all," my client said as she used her rest hours, her leisure time and money to catalog and consolidate the images of their exuberant lives so she could keep those memories with her, organized.

Time to deal with grief before these days arrive may be better than time spent making Goodwill donations after it happens, but of course loss is unpredictable. Sitting with grief is what we do—over the objects, the memories, the lost chances. Family trauma around clutter will exist both while people are alive and after they are gone.

How many homes have I cleaned up after a death? The first one was my childhood home after the death of my parent's marriage—where I watched my mother throw out my dad's things and hide the tapes of our family memories and trips because they were too painful for her to see, let alone watch. Then we cleaned out of my grandmother's apartment when she died—almost too easy because she died with almost nothing left, too stubborn and proud to let her children know she didn't have enough money to buy more food. I remember finding a few packets of ramen noodles and a bag of marshmallows in her cupboard—I ate the noodles and to this day I have the emptied bag of marshmallows saved along with my grandmother's ring. When I feel sad or sick, is it any wonder I reach for the same type of soup she had in her kitchen?

And, of course, cleaning out the closet for my friend and neighbor, mere hours after the police removed his body from the apartment two floors above me, where he died by suicide. Because his husband could no longer look at his things in their shared closet, I was there to help. Crying as we packed up his clothes in a few suitcases and wheeled them out, we removed him entirely and swiftly, just as he had taken himself from our lives. I sobbed as we packed up his things, leaving a half empty closet. I sobbed six months later when my boyfriend packed up his things while I was out on a hike and left our closet half empty also. The death of a relationship and the removal of a half a home's worth of items is hard. When I've helped clients navigate divorce and we separate kitchen tools and children's clothes into two piles to move into new homes, it hurts—even if we all know it is for the best. Any kind of death is a time to pause, reflect, and ask for support from our communities, whether those are friends, chosen family, neighbors, church groups, coworkers, or other social groups.

Decluttering at Home: Reimagining Possibilities

A goal, a vision, an intention—these are similar concepts they resonate differently with people depending on the context. Their similar purpose is helpful though—especially when you are trying to bring a collection of people who live together in a home onto the same wavelength. So pause to define your goals before moving forward.

Now that you have goals, how can you meet them? Setting up a routine can support you to incorporate your goals for your home into your decluttering practice mindfully: mental preparation (priority setting), environment (space cleaning, plants, etc.), physical (movement, food and beverage choices), and connection (with other people, with your passions). Let's move now to some examples of setting up these systems.

My Goals for the Home

Time Needed: 10–15 minutes

Materials Needed: paper, pen, a place to write

Prompt: Read the following passage and write down what comes to mind without censoring yourself. What are the goals, visions, or intentions you have for your home? Set your vision for how you want to feel in your home. For this, use a sentence starter like, "I am a person who . . ." or "In 'x' room, I feel . . ." For example, maybe write, "I am a person who loves where they live" or "In the living room, I feel calm and present with my family." Doesn't that feel good to write?

Consider this as your gata, a mindful mantra to guide your daily activities and your decluttering.

Next, continue exploring the "where." Can you feel at peace here in your home? Write down the places you spend much of your time.

Then move onto the "how." How will you cultivate this feeling? For some people, this may involve burning sage, lighting a candle, opening a window for a breeze, changing the sound (nature frequency), or moving physically in that area.

Now we're at the "what." What will you do to feel decluttered? Maybe it means using sage in your house and setting an intention for what you want to happen and how you want to feel there. For example, do you want to buy less home stuff on your monthly Costco trip? Perhaps you can keep Costco for just food purchases. Get specific here.

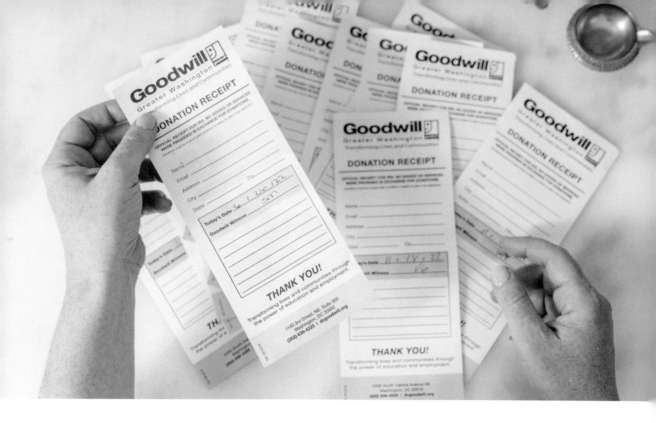

How to Set Up Systems to Declutter Your Home

After we've decluttered the physical things in your home (and set our priorities/goal for how we want to deal with clutter there), we'll make sure everyone who lives and works in the space can maintain the new systems so your vision can flourish. Let's prepare a customized plan to maintain natural organization and flow over time, with written protocols and training to support the desired behavior change and outcome. Plans include schedules for maintenance and the purchasing of household supplies, photos of closet organization, and other established systems unique to your environment. In the health-systems world, we create standard operating practices (SOPs), but here let's call them a systems plan. This is how we can develop the systems you need to get and keep clutter out and monitor the stuff we bring in and our habits/behaviors. All the exercises you've done so far can provide the data and goals you need to translate this work into practice.

Self-Care for the Home (AKA a Maintenance Plan)

Time Needed: 1 hour initially, then several days/weeks/etc.

Materials Needed: paper, pen, a place to write

Directions: Determine who is responsible for which of these tasks across the spectrum of items that live in your environment map.

After completing the earlier exercises, we now have a sense of what our homes look like and volume amounts we want to have to stay within a decluttered home. How are we going to maintain this level of awesomeness? Well let's look closer at the people who are available and responsible for doing different types of things in your home.

Take that environment map and put it to work! What are the habits and maintenance plans needed to keep your home decluttered. Very often they consist of:

- who is buying items;
- who is using them; and
- who is putting them away.

Write down your answers to these questions to set up your maintenance plan. A division of labor for multiple adults who live in a home may be an easy conversation between all parties, or it may require using a tool like Eve Rodsky's *Fair Play* game or a discussion with a therapist to come to agreement. Think about approaching this from a neutral place—

already in this book, you have assessed what the clutter in your home shows up as and set a goal for how you would like your home to be. You know where you would like things to live and how much you want to have. Remove external expectations and self-judgement from these decisions.

Don't make grand proclamations like, "The house will be spotless every night!" Small and achievable next best steps are better for lasting change. Set specific targets like "by when" or "how often should 'x' get done" to maintain the decluttered level you want in your home. Everyone is different in this regard—in my house, our "kind-of-not-totally-dirty" clothing lives on a bench in our bedroom throughout the week until we get to Fridays, which is when I do laundry. I'm OK with this bench and system and urge you to set your own guardrails. If helpful, use calendars or online productivity tools to plot when tasks will get done and by whom.

Decide when you will review how this implementation plan is going. Repetition breeds confidence, so transform the idea of this being a chore into it being a way to feel about living in a decluttered home. Will the review be a time for self-reflection, or would you feel better having it with a coach or as part of a family meeting?

Will you have weekly check-ins? Monthly? What will work best for your home and life? These are good moments to pause, reflect, and make changes if they need to be made. Adaptation is an important part of designing any new system, and the ability to look at this new way of approaching your clutter with an air of curiosity can help encourage positive feelings about it.

Case Study
The House Systems Plan

This is an example of a House Systems Plan, which I laid out for clients of mine in 2021. It brings together their goals for the home, the challenges they had around clutter, and examples of what they could do to mitigate stressors and refresh their space. It also incorporates action steps for them to take toward obtaining and maintaining a mindfully organized home. Use this as a template, if you like, to set goals for your home environment and identify your specific challenges ahead.

GOALS

- To be happy with what we see around us
- To get a handle on the clutter
- To get our home back to feeling as great as it did when we first moved into it
- To have a clear office space that will be better for Zoom calls and productivity
- To maximize the space in our home
- To prepare our home to expand our family

CHALLENGES

- Visual clutter causing stress
- Overwhelmed with items to store
- Lack of closed storage
- Minimal time to maintain order in home

HABIT CHANGES

- Scheduling one hour per week (or two thirty-minute blocks) to put things away
- Maintaining a shopping pause on bringing in anything else new
- Pausing to reflect on whether having the stuff or the space is more important for individual decisions

HOMEWORK

- Purchase hanging folders to complete paperwork task
- Declutter the CD collection, saving only truly special selections or items that cannot be accessed through virtual music libraries

KEY SPACES

Bedroom

- Items to store: clothing, linens, toiletries, dog beds

Suggestions:

- Purchase a wide dresser with proportionally well-sized drawers (not too deep!) to be placed along the wall where current cube system is to better store clothing.

Basement

- Items to store: tools, lightbulbs, DJ equipment, laundry supplies, dog supplies, CDs/tapes, exercise equipment, extra paint

Suggestions:

- Use the extra storage cabinet with doors to contain house tools, lightbulbs, and exercise equipment.
- wall near laundry: pegboard system to hang Swiffer-type items
- Utility closet: store heavy household supplies (i.e., paint) on bottom while shelves above contain lighter household items (i.e., drink dispensers, extra plates).
- Wall near dog crate: use existing storage chest for sentimental CDs/tapes, etc.

Office

- Items to store: desk, clothing, paperwork, books, sentimental items

Suggestions:

- Sell elliptical machine since it is no longer being used.

- Sort books considering these questions: Is this one of your all-time favorite books? Will you read or use this book again?
- Move the cube storage piece from the bedroom into the office and use it to store B's sentimental items, books, and papers.
- Bring a plant into the room now that light is freely flowing into the space.

Main Floor

- Items to store: kitchen supplies, dog supplies and crates, furniture, books, clothing, table with chairs, incoming paperwork

Suggestions:

- Try out this layout option: remove underutilized bookcase (put in upstairs office), move couch closer to corner, and move extra chairs to face couch (creating more defined seating area). The goal is to have comfortable space for sitting and better use of the wall space.

Now that this couple had a plan, the relief on their faces was obvious. There is a saying you may have heard, how "you can't read the label from inside the jar." This couple needed my support—not only to make this plan, but also to reimagine the space altogether. I like to think of them now, selecting a CD they love from their organized music library and finding a comfortable seat on the couch to enjoy the music.

Mindfulness

Mindfulness was just a job to me at first. I felt indignation after leaving my last position at the State Department in the first summer of COVID. The way many colleagues and I had been treated there (with a note that my white able-bodied-ness gave me privilege in that situation of course) upset me. I funneled my rage and eldest-child's need for professional development into a program that seemed perfect for me: a workplace mindfulness facilitator training. I practically shouted into my application, "All of my former workplaces need mindfulness!" thus proving that I, for sure, needed some mindfulness in my own life.

Not new to generic mindfulness practices though, I'd been in plenty of meditation and movement programs that incorporated mindfulness over the years. We also used this extensively in the KonMari Method™ with clients. But thanks to some key core requirements of that training—daily practices, readings, and group work, it was becoming a priority in my life. Great timing, because that Fall I navigated a lot: long delayed housing renovations, a break-in, a wedding. My window of tolerance was barely open.

We've discussed the benefits of mindfulness earlier in this book, but how can we bring that into our homes for decluttering? Consider going through a clearing-space meditation like the one shared on the next page.

Nostalgia

The first time in my adult life that all of my things were in one place was when I was twenty-eight and had recently moved to Swaziland. I had moved from Zambia without a lot of stuff, so I had thousands of pounds available left in my shipment allowance from the State Department. My mother thought this seemed like a great opportunity to have me take ownership back of my childhood artifacts and schoolbooks, which had been taking up space for years in her garage. Thanks, Mom! Included in this shipment were the boxes of T-shirts from soccer tournaments, summers at camp, and other sentimental but not "wear again" shirts for me. They filled several garbage bags, which was an unappealing sight for items I was declaring were important enough to fly across the Atlantic Ocean. Thankfully, around that time, I had heard of T-shirt quilts—probably thanks to an early interest in shelter magazines—and was referred to a seamstress in Swaziland ready to take on the job. I selected my favorite shirts

Mindfulness / Clearing-Space Meditation

Time Needed: 10 minutes

Materials Needed: A quiet place to reflect

Directions: Sit softly on the floor or a chair with your feet planted firmly to feel grounded into the floor. Take a deep breath, hold it for a moment, and then release it softly. We want to create space each day—even if it's just for a moment—for ourselves and our homes. Taking a moment to sit in stillness acts as a simple cleansing for our minds and bodies before we ask them to carry us throughout the day.

Once you are comfortable, read through this scene and let these questions enter your mind to explore what insight they bring.

When you feel ready, imagine yourself walking up to your front door. You feel excited to be home. You imagine all the goodness awaiting you inside.

What makes you feel good in this house?

Breathe in and out, slowly.

You reach for the handle. How does it feel? The door pushes open, and you walk inside.

Imagine it is the most magical moment ever in your home.

Say to yourself, "I live here," with a smile.

Breathe in and out, slowly.

Your favorite scent wafts through the air—what is it?

The lights are set at just the right levels. Are they dim or bright? What do you see around you? How are things laid out?

Breathe in and out, slowly. Picture yourself walking through your space. You move freely; your hands pass over fabrics and objects that feel pleasing to touch.

Picture the ease or energy or beauty that you wish to surround you in your home.

Breathe in and out, slowly.

When you are ready, come out of your mindfulness practice and consider how you can carry those thoughts and energies throughout your day.

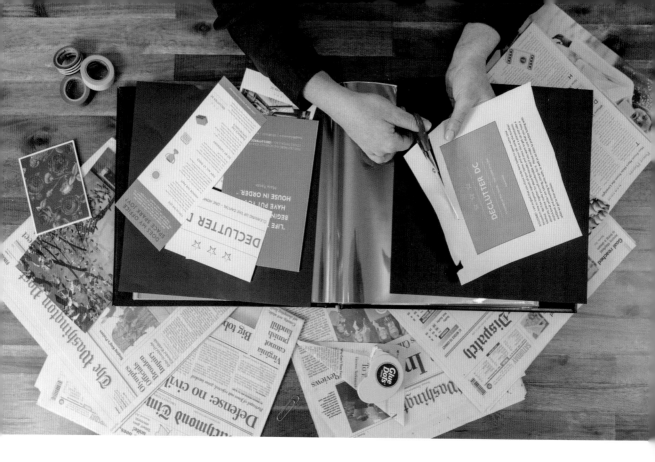

from the bags and donated the ones still in good enough condition to be worn and threw the ones that were essentially rags away. The quilt that this woman made for me in 2009 is a vibrant, joyful, usable piece of nostalgia that I get to cuddle with on the couch whenever I want. It is so much better than leaving items of importance in garbage bags in my mother's garage.

So many people feel like they are not allowed to let go of old papers from their family members, and we have to ask questions that get at why they feel the need to hold onto things. For instance, are you the documentarian for your family? If so, are you holding onto items in a way that allows you to tell those stories easily and with compassion, like displaying a photo album with special collected memories, or does the volume/weight of the items/clutter weigh you down so much that instead of enjoying the storytelling experience, you resent it? Boxes and boxes of family heirlooms and photos and collections can do this. The client I mentioned ear-

Creatively Editing Nostalgia

Time Needed: 10 minutes (more time later for creating your project)

Directions: Think about how you would like to experience nostalgia at home.

Which items do you have the most difficulty parting with? For many people, these are sentimental items (often photos or letters), so how can we create art based on the artifacts around us? If going through nostalgic items is hard for you, you're not alone. One mindfulness technique would be to use your five senses while going through nostalgic items and deciding what to keep based on what positively activates your senses. Consider the following.

- What smells do you like to have around you?
- Are there things you like to see that bring you joy?
- What colors inspire good feelings?
- Are the photographs you want to keep telling your story, the one you want to be able to share and live and use?
- Are there sounds that make you happy, like playing or listening to music?
- Are there foods you enjoy eating?
- Are there fabrics you like to touch?

Use which senses and memories have come to mind during this reflection. As you wade through the nostalgia in your home look for examples of these experiences and memories to come forth. Do they start to form stories about moments from your past that are pleasant? If so, keep note of those to use when creating experiences that honor them in your home. Albums, collages, shadow boxes are all examples of how these items can be experienced at home. You may find other ways that are singular to your life, and your home that resonate for you to create.

lier, whose mother had thousands and thousands of bells, would become overwhelmed with what to do next when she looked at her large collection. We started slowly and brought a few of the bells home—it was the holiday season, so we deliberately took a few holiday-themed ones. Then she gave some of them away as gifts to family friends who wanted them. Relief and enjoyment started to rise when she could see how she didn't need the whole collection to remember her mother's interest, which then helped her loosen her attachment to the overall volume of the collection.

Items in a home can be important tools to bring out our self-identity. They make our homes feel like *home*. But when there are too many items—or the items breed stress and negativity—they detract from our feelings of home. Nostalgia turns into a burden in moments like these.

When people feel out of control in their lives or their homes, they may cling to nostalgia or nostalgic memories of things because it helps them feel as though they're back in a time they remember (either correctly or not) as being happy or calm. These feelings can be corrupted to influence others. Take former president Trump's rhetoric around "Make America Great Again" as an example of nostalgia tainted from his viewpoint.

Simon Sinek's book ***Start with Why*** offers insight into values and nostalgia. Every brand with an online presence has been increasing their amount of advertising while fighting for our attention and money, which is also our loyalty. No wonder we feel overwhelmed to buy and keep things—because so many more of the brands or types of items we are purchasing have been imbued with a sense of collegiality or comradeship with the item itself. When I was decluttering my closet, I thought, *How can I get rid of my M.M.LaFleur pants? They're such a great company. I love them and I identify with them—letting go of those pants would be the loss of identity.*

Our things become markers for the symbols of ideas we hold dear, and so decluttering those objects tells our brain that somehow, we have forsaken those ideals and/or we are no longer part of the club of like-minded people who buy and use them. This is an identity crisis.

Reframing our experience with nostalgic items may help with this crisis. We know that creativity is a vital part of being healthy humans, families, and communities. How can we use creativity to transform nostalgic clutter at home into well-being opportunities?

Consider incorporating art into your home as a memory-management tool during your decluttering. This can cultivate joy (by activating positive neuroaesthetics of your home) while respecting your home (by downsizing the volume of stuff creating clutter). This also makes it easier to share your stories and nostalgic items with others (connection). We've explored neuroaesthetics a bit so far. Let's revisit it as a practice.

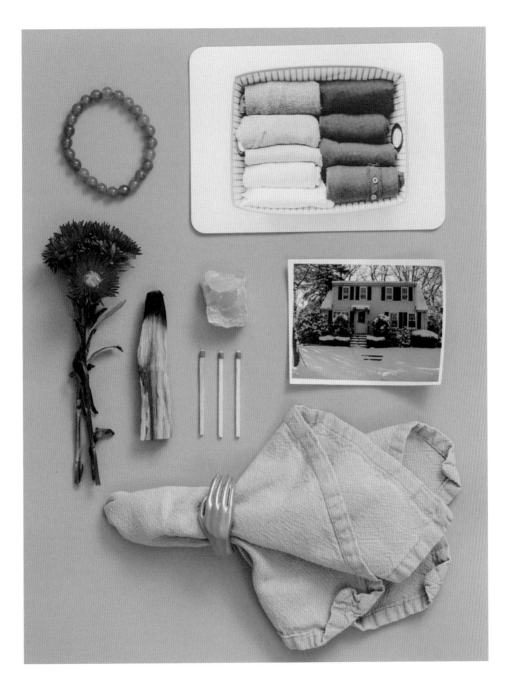

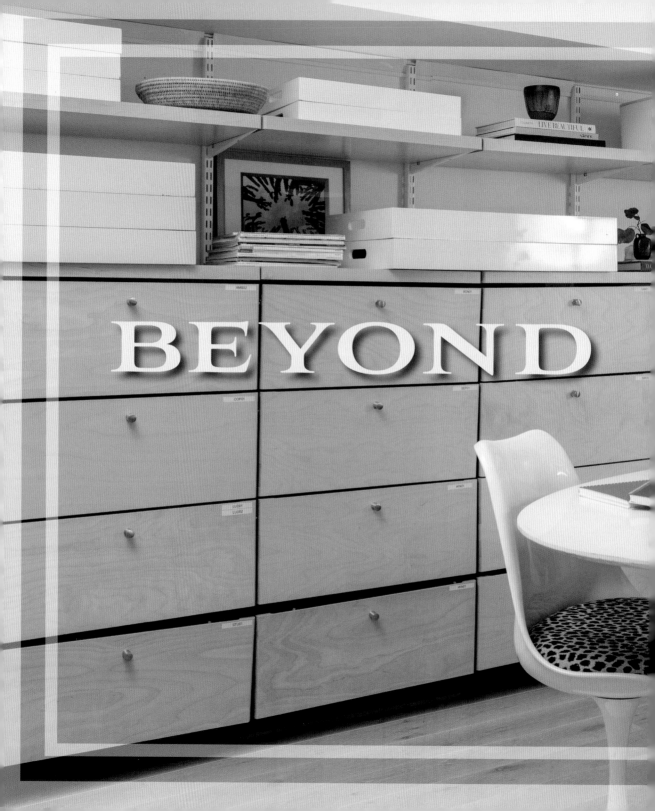

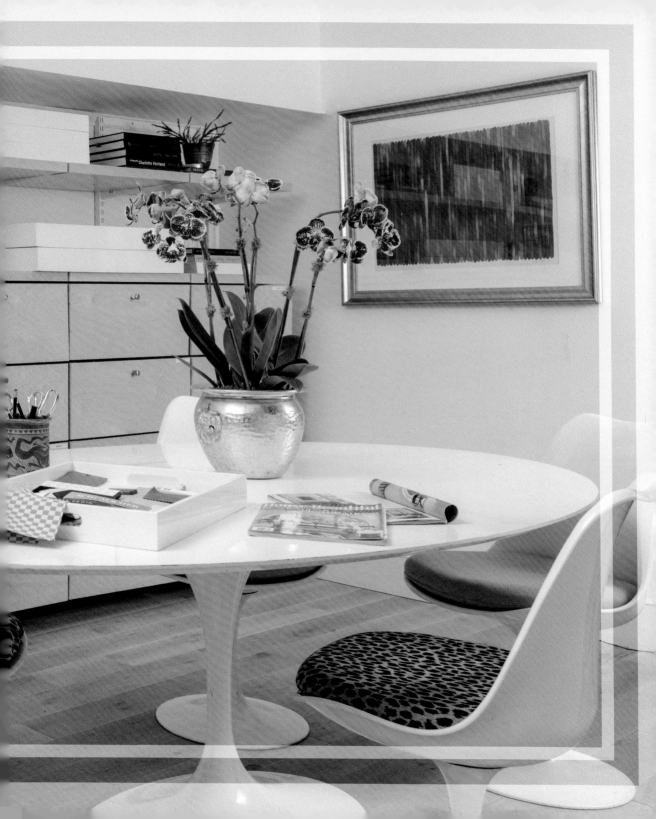

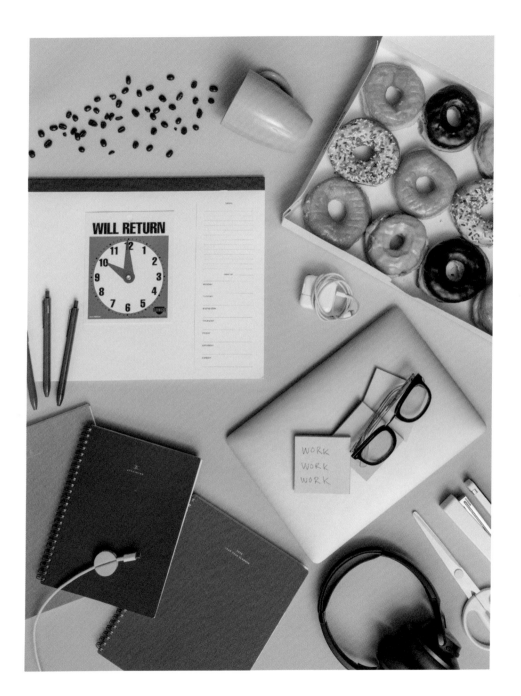

BEYOND

I once worked for a program where the mission was palpable, and the tensions ran high. Our office, where a hive of fifty dedicated and frantic public health officials fought over budgets and politics in the name of global health, was in a beige stucco building two blocks from the White House. Whatever effort was made was never enough, personally or for the cause—for instance, after five years of working in this program, someone I knew resigned and was accused of "not caring about people with AIDS" anymore because "how dare she put her own well-being above that of the program's beneficiaries." Shortly after she left, we received an office satisfaction survey and—shocker—the results were grim. People reported low morale, little hope, and dwindling concern for the mission. The utmost care had been taken with services to be provided for beneficiaries of the program, with barely any compassion shown for those of us working on it. The volume and visibility of the issues was becoming too overwhelming to ignore and I speculated about what reactionary changes would happen next to quell the grumbling uprising upon us.

What was the first thing leadership did to raise spirits? They brought donuts to the office on Fridays. And they didn't just bring them in and leave them in the lunchroom; they brought them in and had the office secretary send an all-staff email to *announce* that leadership had brought in said donuts in a "wow how wonderful that our big boss deigned to bring us donuts" tone. Each time the email arrived in my inbox, I sighed at the hypocrisy—because, yes, I was absolutely going to eat one, and, no, this was not actually solving anything. This performative gift continued every week with the same two boxes of donuts, the same exclamatory email, and wow, donuts again! Meanwhile, burnout spread through the cubicles as scopes of work were stretched beyond limits and offers of sugary treats came in the place of right-sized performance expectation.

I remember sitting at my desk one day, munching on half of a glazed donut and wondering if I'd gotten to a place in my organizing business where I had enough financial security to resign from gaslighting central. Calculating that by April, the next month, I would be on a trajectory to cover my financial responsibilities with what I earned in my business, I set my path toward resigning. The leadership model I had seen throughout my government career was so different than what I was trying to embody as my own business owner and the disconnect in my feelings was causing ambivalence towards the mission of my work (something that didn't feel good). Plus, I could certainly afford my own donuts when I wanted them.

As I signed contracts for corporate presentations to be delivered in person over the next few weeks, I felt like I could finally declutter my financial ties to the office. I had a waiting list of in-person clients and was ready to be done with cubicle life and spend more time in their closets. It was March of 2020, and the possibilities ahead were exciting.

Underlying Issues

Weekly donuts may be delicious, but in my experience, they do not solve any root problems of workplace tension. Tension pops up at work when priorities are always changing, or when there is some combination of too many decision makers, unfair hiring and payment practices, and unrealistic to-do lists (among other things of course). These are some examples of disorganization in a workplace because they represent behaviors and environments that can accumulate and affect our well-being. And it's not just workplaces where this happens—problematic behaviors and environments can surround us online or in real life beyond apartments and offices. That's why I titled this chapter "Beyond"—because I wanted to set aside room for you to consider how mindful organizing can be applied to other environments where you spend your time. Here we'll discuss clutter in the context of personal and professional goals.

It's also why I think it's not just homes that benefit from decluttering with a holistic perspective. Wherever we are spending our time and whatever occupies our life deserve mindful attention. There is more to declutter in our lives than just our closets. To figure out what that is, we must go deeper into the beyond, teasing out our underlying mission for what we want out of life and creating systems that allow us to move closer to alignment with those goals. Let's dive in.

Disorganized environments and behaviors can impact our well-being in many ways—but we don't have to accept this. Typically, the overwhelming feelings I've seen people grapple with beyond their homes and health issues can be broken down into three categories, not mutually exclusive but certainly overlapping and helpful to organize for our purposes:

- Work
- Ideas
- Connections

Work

Even before I began my career as an adult, my passion was clear: I wanted to throw my professional energy into global HIV/AIDS programs. I started volunteering in local HIV/AIDS organizations in Boston during middle school, when my uncle succumbed to the disease. By the end of college, the epidemic was rapidly spreading in Africa so I headed across the Atlantic to join the response efforts there. I studied international public health in graduate school, and from 2003 onward, I traveled around the globe for the PEPFAR. It was impactful. It was rewarding. It was exhausting.

After thirteen years of travel, I settled into what was supposed to be the "right" position for where I was in my life and career: midlevel management at a government agency in Washington, DC, where I tackled the issues I was deeply passionate about—except I didn't feel that passion anymore. Surrounding me were some of the most negative people I had ever encountered, and it began to affect my outlook on every aspect of the job. On paper, everything looked good—maybe even great—but my days were mind-numbing. I spent hours wasting time writing emails in support of programs I didn't believe in but had to advocate for so we wouldn't lose our budget. Short and shallow breaths were the soundtrack in my office as I reviewed the legal hurdles of bureaucracy to try to remove staff members making egregious errors. I was at a loss about what to do.

How could I feel this way about a program I'd once been so passionate about?

I figured if I worked harder, I could overcome the doubt that I was making any difference anymore—the strategy backfired. I grew insecure, thinking I had made the wrong choice in taking this job, and feared I had to stay in it because I was supposed to be grateful for the role, the leadership, the salary. I put in longer hours, stress-ate Chex Mix at my desk, and let my exercise habits slide along with my mood. I no longer saw a future in my chosen field, which never looked like anything other than miserable, but I felt too far along to do anything about it.

I was burned out. This was way before the World Health Organization (WHO) had recognized burnout in 2019 as a medical condition resulting from chronic workplace stress that has not been successfully managed. I didn't know it, but I was having a physiological response to having too many problems and priorities at work and not enough resources to manage them. Resources could include money (to hire people to do some of the tasks I was assigned) or even rest (the ability for my body to repair itself in between moments of stress) but what if these resources weren't available or even widely known? I felt like a cog in a wheel—and the wheel was splintering.

Stressful work environments are not a new concept. Nor should they be a given way of working. Thoughtfully interrogating what is causing the stress and then decluttering (reducing, removing, or reallocating the points of contention) is important. Like I introduced in the health chapter, disciplines like workplace sociology offer a framework for unpacking these situations by asking questions like, "How do we create the environments that support corporate goals and offer sustainable solutions so that people can thrive?" Now that the world has reached crescendo levels of burnout, mental health challenges, and economic crises alongside levels of awareness of these problems, it would be great if that awareness could translate into action. Workplaces could finally start doing the mindful decluttering and organizing needed to mitigate the harm to well-being being caused by that stress.

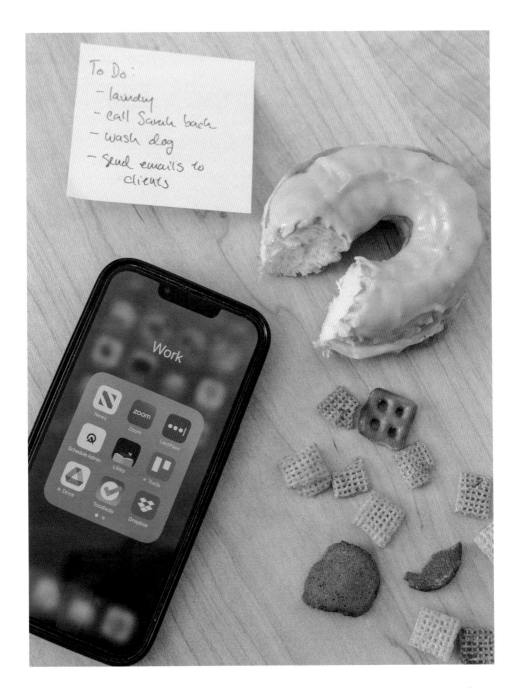

To Do:
- laundry
- call Sarah back
- wash dog
- send emails to
  clients

One source of stress can be the environment where work is happening. A confined cubicle farm, with a hierarchy of closed doors. A place where invites to meetings are doled out like runway tickets. Login codes to conference calls are a closely held secret. Information guarded, protected, hidden. Oh sorry, just my former workplaces? Of course, work lends itself to negativity when clouded within such a setup. With so much drama around how people are treating each other we may get distracted from looking at some of the basic infrastructure around us: is there any sunlight near me? Am I breathing in toxins? Like environmental health concerns in a home, there are aspects to think about for work environments also. Circle back to the home chapter where I shared the environmental health concerns to take note of and consider how these are monitored in your work environment.

Like the creativity exercise for environmental mapping of your home suggested in chapter two, what would you find if you applied that same lens to your work environment? Could you bring in these eight categories to investigate whether or not where you spend your time working (that could be at home, in a local coffee shop or an office setting—however you define work and where it takes place matters here?

Once we have a good handle on these key environmental factors around us, the container where we are existing, let's take some time to examine what is taking up space in this place. The stuff does matter in a workplace. Physical clutter here can cause actual harm, like in situations where exit doors get blocked by a build-up of old equipment thus presenting a fire hazard. These are important factors to be aware of, and standards set by organizations like the Occupational Safety and Health Administration (OSHA) offer guidelines for safety to protect people in certain industries and workplaces. Awareness of and adhering to these guidelines can be protective.

Very often when workplaces assess their clutter, they focus on items that fall into physical products, papers, or digital documents. But clutter at work is not always about a messy mail pile on a desk. It's also about stressful psychological or structural conditions. Structural issues here are largely a volume issue—too many tasks for too few people to complete, for instance— whereas psychological issues are underlying or confounding circumstances. An example of psychological clutter could be when there are unclear expectations of what must be done, by when, and to what standard. There are so many possibilities, and you may not know which one leads to the outcomes or goals you want to achieve. This is closely tied to technological clutter, such as not being sure where your documents are in a computer or a cloud system that is full. Devices clogged with out-of-date screenshots or voice memos can impair their ability to operate and your ability to focus on the work you most want to do, and may leave you susceptible to fraud/phishing schemes because you are too bogged down to stay aware of potential threats.

For most adults, a significant amount of our focus is placed on our work lives, which may be paid or unpaid labor efforts—it's up to you to define that—but regardless, work can be full of situations and experiences causing stress (i.e., the clutter at work). The last two-plus decades of working in the global health sphere brought me in touch with hundreds of highly committed colleagues—people who are working to advance economic, educational, and health services for neighbors, friends, and strangers around the world. Over time and in many different countries, I experienced firsthand the personal strain that type of work can have on people. I saw the way burnout and stress can eat at our compassion and our resilience, especially when we work within challenging systems.

Some companies and industries are taking notice of this stress and supporting studies on its impact on the workforce. For instance, Deloitte reports that 77 percent of workers experience burnout. The current global climate is full of women leaving the workforce in droves while companies scramble to hire and retain committed employees. While I'm glad to see more awareness of the rising diagnosed rates of ADHD and menopause symptoms, the sad truth is that they undermine women's abilities to work as they would like to, affecting their workplace outputs as well. Underlying health issues follow us throughout our lives no matter what types of work we do.

While employees gain a greater sense of personal balance and productivity, companies benefit from a more efficient, energized team advancing the organization toward its goals. Workplaces can adopt techniques to improve employee satisfaction and retention by creating and implementing sustainable methods for workspace organization. Decluttering can be a container for our transformation within our work spheres. To do that, you first need to assess where you are.

Becoming increasingly mindful about specific issues at work that influence your experience will allow you to act in the right direction and address them. This awareness is a form of workplace mindfulness, which when endorsed and promoted can help organizations address

Journaling on Our Work Clutter

Time Needed: 15 minutes

Materials Needed: Something to write with (pen, pencil, marker) and something to write in (journal, notebook—something with enough room to write in a few times)

Prompt: How can we determine where clutter shows up for us in our work lives?

Instructions: Move through the list of questions and write down what comes to mind without censoring yourself. Answer these questions as truthfully as you can.

During your journaling session, give yourself a quiet space to write and think. Spend at least three minutes reflecting on each of the following questions.

- What comes up when you think of work?
- What emotions or memories came up when you read the story about my former workplace at the start of this chapter?
- Regarding burnout and stress affecting clutter at work, can you think of any examples of how that shows up for people you know (or for yourself)?
- Describe a way someone struggling with clutter at work could be supported by other people.
- Is there anything else you want to write about clutter and work that I haven't asked you about yet?

loneliness, anxiety, and burnout by establishing a connection between team members and a healthy workplace culture where individuals can grow and flourish as part of a team.

Ideas

Piles of articles littered his bed, each with a sticky note promising prestige and notoriety. The next journal submission! The next contract! It was all possible if only the articles and scraps of paper could meld into fully formed deliverables without requiring any of Peter's time and attention. If only.

His forehead crinkled with concern, as though I had come to snatch his articles (and thus his future) away from him. Our discussion about letting go of some of the older notes and articles on topics now out of date did not go well. "But what if I need this someday?" he pleaded as though I was physically trying to take them away from him.

(Reader, I was not, in fact, physically trying to take these pages away from him.)

Reason did not exist in that moment to keep all these papers, not with the magic of the internet providing current and easily accessible information on a variety of topics, and certainly not with his priorities for time management. He was a busy legal partner and soon a new father—and this collection of articles representing new work to do would stay part of his daily life if he didn't change. Clinging to the ideas and possibilities in the boxes full of notes and paper scraps, he treated them like a sacred baby blanket from childhood, giving them priority in his house over the growing pile of incoming supplies for the actual baby due to arrive the next month.

Peter's resistance to decluttering seemed more focused on me and my ideas than on what he had hired me for—to declutter his own ideas, the hundreds of them now sorted on his blue bedspread. His larger resistance to change and letting go of papers came in part from not trusting himself to remember the ideas or citations when they might be needed. The resistance to start the next big idea or article or paper was strong and closely tied to shame around not having completed the project yet, or not knowing if he'd ever be able to start it. I know I could relate to aspects of that resistance while writing this book. I had so many ideas and concepts for what would be helpful to include, and ultimately, had to decide what made the best sense *right now*—for **this** book, in **this** moment. To delay it any longer for how the next idea could potentially improve some section was doing a disservice to this book and its readers.

More so than any torn sweaters or college textbooks, the clutter of ideas cause some of the greatest challenges for people I work with. We are extrapolating a bit here—in my field, I expand the idea of clutter to go beyond the items strewn about in a disorganized fashion. Yes, in general, clutter is a collection of items people accumulate in their homes and don't necessarily use but hold on to anyway. But I am fascinated by how our very thoughts, dreams, and ideas can be cluttered too; I think this area has been overlooked for too long. Jumbles of possibilities, locked in our brains, as messy as overstuffed closets. And perhaps even more distracting.

Cluttered ideas may show up physically—scrap papers with thoughts of books to look up or articles to write—or they might be digitally stuffed into your phone—seventy-five tabs open to things to buy or read, plus all those voice notes you dictated to yourself while driving that you didn't want to forget. (Hi! That's my favorite container for ideas.)

Our ideas represent an abundance of possibility, knowledge that is exciting yet unmanaged. And it may feel positive in one sense—"I have so many ideas for stories to write!"—but when there are that many to think about and you can't separate out the good ones from the bad, the feeling of abundance can become overwhelming. This happens when ideas are unorganized, underused, and on their way to metabolizing into guilt or anxiety—"Look at all these ideas I haven't touched, I feel useless!"

But so often time goes by and ideas stack up. We move forward, interested in new things and doing new things. The ideas sit and the pile grows.

It can be hard to let go of ideas because they might represent unfulfilled plans or desires. For people with ADHD, there may be a fear of getting rid of ideas because they have learned not to trust themselves over the years when their symptoms were not being managed and they might have had experiences forgetting or misplacing things that needed to be done. Ideas tend to pile up when our minds are always racing with too many ideas to implement without time being spent acting on them.

For clothing, we may know that we should put it away in a closet or a dresser, but ideas are nebulous. Where should they live? How will I find them again? How many is the right amount

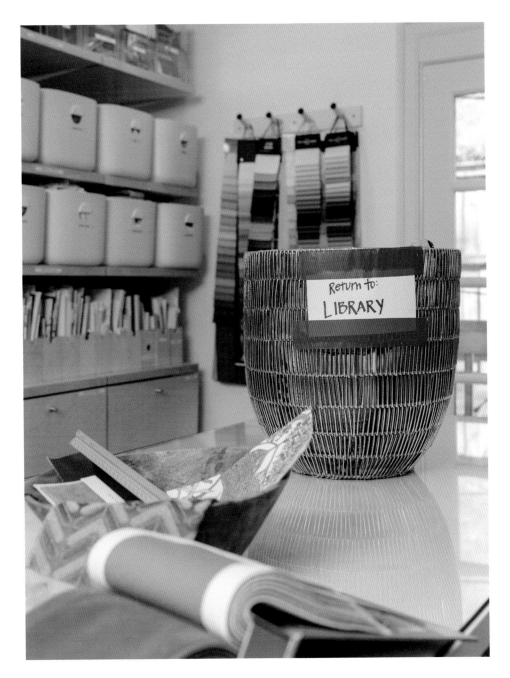

Return to:
LIBRARY

to keep? Managing knowledge is a skill set that deserves some attention upfront to save you time in the long run—much like setting up a closet or pantry system.

Social media and living in a connected world bring us a constant stream of information and ideas. Platforms repeatedly offer us new ways of thinking about things and options for what to do. Being presented with new information is wonderful if you can harness it to improve your life, but too much of a good thing results in a surplus of options and stress about which things are truly worthy of our time and attention.

To begin to declutter our ideas, let's make sure we can first locate them.

Make a Home for Your Ideas

Today there is no shortage of online or physical keepers for recording ideas, intentions, tasks, and goals. Very rarely is one place the right option for all things. You might like Evernote for organizing your to-read articles but not your to-do list. That's OK. Don't let perfect be the enemy of good enough. Try to find a balance between not using anything and using too many systems. Most of our phones and technology also have options for recording information and calendarizing tasks, which are the principal functions we need.

Above all, we want to make these ideas accessible. Can you readily find what you put on a list? Electronic platforms make this easier, especially if you move around to different places in your day, week, or life, and you need to access this info from different areas. The search bar works wonders. Notebooks with labeled sections are also good if you adhere to regularly opening, using, and checking them.

Think about what came up in your assessment of clutter in your work life. What types of ideas came up? Are they actions to take or knowledge to manage? Knowing what you do about how it presents itself and the amount of time it takes from your life, what aspects do you want to address?

This is why I remind my clients that decluttering is more than getting the right containers for your home. Mindfully organized containers for our ideas are also critical on a decluttering journey. It's a daily decision to welcome increased flow, joy, and presence into your life. The next

Where Do Your Ideas Live?

Time Needed: 15 minutes

Materials Needed: Something to write with (pen, pencil, marker) and something to write in (journal, notebook—something with enough room to write in a few times)

Instructions: Move through the list of questions below and write down what comes to mind without censoring yourself. Answer these questions as truthfully as you can.

- Which ideas represent your priorities right now?
- Do you feel comfortable knowing what to do next?
- Do you have a way to store and access ideas you need to act on?
- Do you know how you want to feel when you look for and use your ideas?
- How much time do you want to spend putting your ideas into action?

Responses to these questions can help craft your plan for how to store and use your ideas.

exercise will help you bring awareness to the types of ideas cluttering your life and how you want to use them.

Many times, the ideas we cling to are less about the items and more about what loss they represent. I kept years' worth of professional ideas stacked in a closet in my last home reminding me of what I gave up.

When I left my office job in 2016, I brought home a giant stack of training manuals, reference materials, and publications I had produced. I carried from desk to desk over the course of more than a decade working in global health. As I was applying the KonMari Method™ to my papers, I held onto them as a "just for when" moment—that time *when* I would head back to an office, or another similar job, and need them again. I was sure that *when* moment would eventually come.

That stack of manuals sat in my coat closet for years, tucked off to the side, on the two lower shelves of a bookcase that I had been carting around since I'd left Zambia in 2008. Out of the corner of my eyes as I would reach in to grab a jacket or put one away, I'd half see them, never focusing on them fully but also never forgetting they were there. One April, I remembered this dormant pile and thought, *Is it when yet?* I'd just started a new global health assignment, so I took a closer look at these materials—and you know what? I didn't need 95 percent of them. And for the few that might have been relevant, I found better, updated examples and publications online. I saved my favorite pieces from the pile—the best examples of work that I am proud of—and recycled or shredded the rest. Perhaps a bit wistful in the moment, but I didn't dwell on that or scold myself for making the decision to let go of them. I didn't want to ask myself if it was *when* yet for the next twenty years and torture myself with decision paralysis. It turned out my "just for when" papers had been a "just in case" collection that I was probably having a hard time letting go of after my last job because it had been such a big life change for me. Years later, I was ready to let go, not only of the papers but of that exhausting, hopeful, stressful, and semichaotic part of my life. I embraced the idea that who I used to be was allowed to feel better about who I am *now*. Decluttering invites external and internal transformations like this.

The next week, after reducing this bulk of stuff, I found myself more energized around the home. Having made the decision that *when* was *now*, it was easier to work on my new assignment and get excited about the current information I could dig into. With two shelves emptied of the stories from my past, I now had much more space to think, plan, and give ideas for my future room to develop.

Having that space gave me mental clarity on what was important. In the same way I encourage people to practice wearing some of their clothing that doesn't get worn regularly, you should also practice using some of the ideas that are taking up space. Take baby steps. Is there an article you have been meaning to write? Dedicate thirty minutes to starting it. Today. A pile of knitting on the floor? Assign it to yourself as homework on Friday evenings, when you need to unplug anyway. And if it feels like you aren't quite ready to start doing these things, make sure they are listed in your Ideas Home or on your someday/maybe list. An Ideas Home can be a physical or digital space. Some people like corkboards for pinning to-do lists, dream ideas, and monthly goals. Other people have a simple file on their computer where they track various ideas. Wherever your Ideas Home is, treat it as a space that needs decluttering every now and then, just like the closet. Our habits need a home too, or at least a place where we track them. Remember that someday/maybe list from the previous chapter? This kind of organizational tool can help us align our actions with our values and remember what is important. It's a way to increase our awareness *before* we click "purchase." Which is important given the ease of online spending and targeted ads that compel us to buy more stuff with diminishing returns and satisfaction.

Connections

How does clutter show up in our connections? When the volume of time and the quality of the interactions are not positively influencing our lives. This can be seen when too much time spent on social media leads to mental health problems. Or when too little time and quality of social interactions drives the epidemic of loneliness and isolation in the United States.

Connections within and outside of our homes, families, and workplaces are critical for our well-being. Enhancing our firsthand experiences of mindfulness enables us to better understand and then choose how to design meaningful connections. Building pauses into your day for reflection, for rest, allows this type of mindfulness to begin affecting your nervous system. Pauses are vital for our health. We only need ninety seconds, for example, to identify a strong emotion and let it flow through our body, according to Harvard brain scientist Dr. Jill Bolte Taylor. But usually within that ninety-second window, we reach for our phone or remote, suppressing the emotion rather than identifying it and letting it rise and fall. Even a few minutes of resting your eyes while sitting up or taking a short walk outside with no external distractions (e.g., podcasts in your headphones) can add to your cup of mindfulness. Increasing our mindfulness allows us to be less reactive to ideas and stressors that come up. In a world where productivity is seen as a virtue, taking an occasional pause might feel like a radical act. To reclaim her free time and encourage others to do the same, artists and filmmaker Tiffany Shlain, author of *24/6: The Power of Unplugging One Day a Week,* advocates for unplugging from technology one day a week. While not everyone can do that, is there one small change you can make where you can add a pause in your day?

When we talk about mindfulness within a work environment, we think about how we can be with ourselves and others in our organizations, aligned by shared values and mission. Although I am not advocating for connection to become a productivity-driven and measured

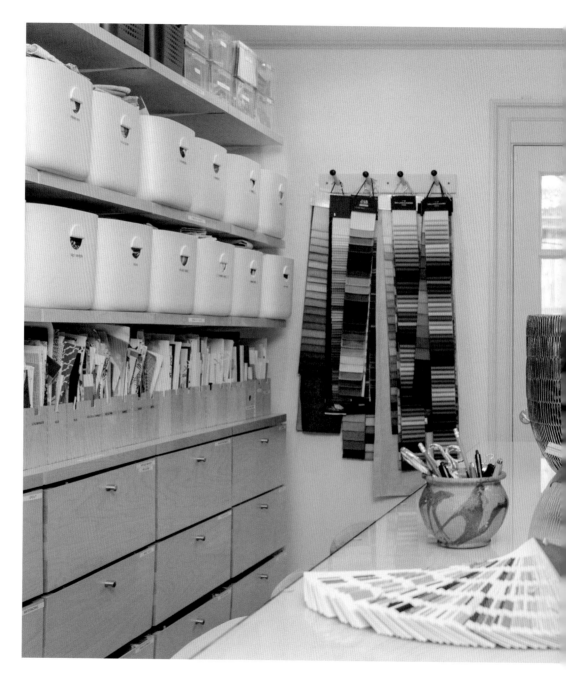

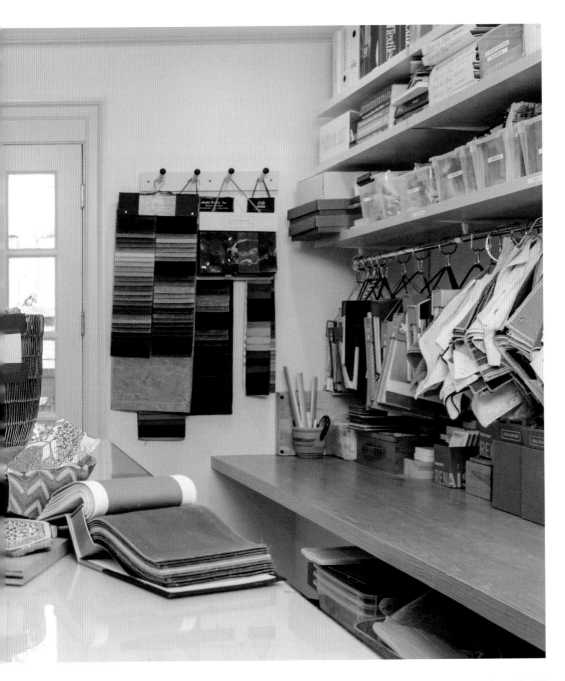

must-do within a work culture, it is necessary, especially if this is new for your group, to build in time for this to occur. This space and time allow people to become aware of the connections around them—what feels overwhelming versus nourishing.

Aside from our homes and our jobs, our relationships with other people have a tremendous impact on our well-being. When we connect with people who do not share our values or interests, we have cluttered our attention and time. Often people are afraid to declutter their relationships because they think of the sunk costs, such as the time they have already allocated to those relationships, and how it can be hard to make new connections. But our social surroundings influence our thoughts and actions, so if they are not aligned with our intentions, we are moving in the wrong direction.

During my twenties, my relationship with my father grew more and more painful to maintain. I tried to stay present and participate in a relationship with him, because I clung to the idea that since this was my father, I had to, that this was ostensibly a connection I needed to maintain above all. But after years of pain and disappointment, it finally took a conversation with my friend Jeremy, who said, "You've tried very hard, and you don't have to keep trying anymore if it doesn't feel good," for me to feel like I had permission to let that relationship go. And, of course, it wasn't that I felt I needed Jeremy's permission in that moment—but I needed to be seen and heard by someone who could help me acknowledge that I had a choice and that I did not have to remain in something that was hurting me.

This type of discussion, permission, and weighing of our choices around the most problematic and raw parts of life calls on so much personal awareness. I'm reminded of how Jeremy helped me with this decision about my father over and over in client sessions when I sit with people, listen, and offer them permission to declutter connections that are painful and irresolvable.

Besides helping people assess relationships in their life, friends can also show allyship for people who are dealing with overwhelming situations; you can do even without being a professional organizer. It is a beautiful element of true friendship, or even respectful collegiality. Our connections (outside of family) may include friends, colleagues, and community groups of all kinds. How can we use connection to help our loved ones and people in our communities? Consider exploring these examples and locating one or two options that could be tried out in one of your communities:

- Educational institutions are showing signs of increasing attention on wellness. Temple University has canceled classes on Fridays for people to be able to focus on wellness. Virginia Tech is building out a digital well-being program with *The Joy of Missing Out (JOMO)* author Christina Crook. Decluttering within these community spaces complements educational goals under these wellness programs.

- Tricia Hersey's Nap Ministry recommends communal rest and dream gatherings that center black liberation and offer space to use rest to resist systemic oppression (as detailed in her book of the same name). Her work positions rest as a right, and the ability to rest as needed—particularly in connection with others—is enough on its own and helps people feel more mindful in their lives.

- Tiffany Shlain advocates for a schedule where at least one day a week, we are "off" from technology, work, etc. Her book *24/6: Giving Up Screens One Day a Week to Get More Time, Creativity, and Connection* offers plenty of great ideas.

- In some companies, sick days are being rebranded as "wellness" days or allowing for ad hoc mental health days. If you are in management or admin, remember that if wellness does not include opportunities to reflect on different aspects of clutter, you are ignoring baseline concerns that also lead to health problems.

- Some offices set goals as a group and track progress together, just like gold-star charts in elementary school or a thermometer with meditation or mindful minutes/moments. Anything that counts as innovative and connective team-building exercises (ones that center compassion, connection, and resiliency) can be useful here, provided that they are optional events.

Decluttering the Beyond: Lead with Clarity

She eyed the stack of boxes filled with impeachment files and sighed. *Are we really doing this?* her eyes said as she looked my way. *Oh heck yes.* I smiled back, finally at a prized category after months of ordinary paper sorting and discarding in other rooms. She knew it had to happen eventually, so she hefted one of the higher boxes down to the ground and pulled off the top. Thirty boxes in a row are intimidating to start with but not as intimidating as the trial itself, I imagined. Each box that we opened gave us a glimpse into the past, a historic moment at the time,

Assess Potential Cluttered Connections

Time Needed: 15 minutes

Materials Needed: pencil/pen, paper

Prompt: Where are cluttered relationships manifesting in your life?

Instructions: Spend three minutes each writing down your responses to the following:

- Are there people in your life who consistently make you feel great and with whom you'd love to spend more time connecting?

- Which people in your life, if any, are consistently hurting you? Or people you always feel terrible or drained after seeing or calling them?

- What comes up for you for when you think about your connection to these people?

- Are there any goals you have for connection in your life?

- Is there a local volunteer or hobby group that might attract people with similar values or interests as you?

By reducing the attention and time spent in relation with people who bring out negative feelings of connection, there is more opportunity for authentic relationships.

though now little more than your average decade-plus paperwork. I thought of all the recent news stories of misplaced government files as I grabbed a box filled with binders of paperwork that I quickly pulled apart. As she opened each box, her face relaxed a bit and her *hmmms* grew gentler. "OK shred. This is unsealed material now, so I don't need to keep it," she said about the first box. And the next and the next and the next. The stack against the wall grew smaller with only the occasional "oh wow I remember this speech" bringing some levity to the otherwise dusty garage and the paper being placed into a small "keep" pile in the corner. Initially thrilled to go through such legendary material, I eventually grew bored with the endless copies of transcripts needing to be shredded and started quickly ripping through the boxes marked "sealed with sensitive material." Even better, she moved quickly now too. Usually only proud of herself for bills passed or policies enacted, today was different. The pile was being shredded away, and a feeling of relief was growing. Her past no longer waited for her in a suburban garage.

Clutter affects everyone and when it is weighing down those in leadership positions, that stress can trickle down to others. As mental health challenges and awareness of them have grown, leaders can no longer claim ignorance of the multidimensional experiences of people around them. This is true for workplaces, faith-based organizations, and other community networks. How leaders lead has an impact on the well-being of others—something that wasn't a concern for my first boss in Zambia, who used to send emails in ALL CAPS when she was mad about something.

Individual bosses and how they talk to staff can go a long way in making people feel appreciated. More managers are understanding the importance of addressing mental health at work and learning how to integrate attention to employees' mental well-being in their own leadership practices. Eighty-eight percent of HR professionals believe that offering mental health benefits can boost productivity, and 86 percent think it helps with employee retention.

Workplaces can create a positive impact on employee well-being, and this can include leaders buying in to the idea that decluttering is critical, knowing that this is not an either-or situation. Workplaces that identify a champion to integrate decluttering into the culture may have greater long-term success with changing how people feel at work.

Are you an employer who wants to create a system that allows your staff to operate with less overwhelm? Establishing a mindful and compassionate work environment and the practices to sustain it can help transform professional spaces. Workplaces can create a positive impact on employee well-being. This can include leaders buying into the need that decluttering is critical. It may help to identify a champion in your office who can help to integrate this into culture.

If you've finished the exercises in the previous sections of this chapter, then you've created specific goals and determined the volume and quantity of clutter in your life. Nice! Now let's prepare for the next part: getting the support we need from ourselves, our families, and our communities.

Mindful Support

Since 2017 I've been offering workshops on decluttering topics to companies. It started by sharing about the KonMari Method™—the book and Netflix show brought decluttering to the mainstream and people were excited to learn more about implementing Marie's method, so it's a great way to dive in. Over time, as my awareness of opportunities decluttering can offer, I began teaching sessions on a broader range of topics. Where it gets tricky with workplace lessons is knowing if actual, sustained change for their environments. But some companies are at least trying out those changes, and guess what? Their staff are happier, more fulfilled, and more focused during the workday. It's a start.

Sometimes I was booked for workplace sessions through corporate wellness groups. Groups like these offer opportunities for the companies they support to foster connectivity and well-being for their staff through virtual and on-site offerings. Through them, I've learned that companies want to combat burnout and boost employee health and happiness. Support can arrive in the shape of on-site massages or acupuncture or workshops like the ones I teach on mindfulness and structuring healthy workdays. Even general, fun connection activities, like group trivia, can foster connection among teammates. These umbrella companies, with a roster of service providers like myself, help provide a menu of options employees can choose from based on their needs and wants. Lots of employees, it turns out, want professional decluttering help.

Although the rise in working from home has benefits for many people and companies, it can also cause some malaise (being in the same place all day every day) and disconnection (from a lack of colleagues and in-office working culture). Companies that are proactively trying to enhance their employees' morale in these situations often look for fun ways to break up the day or escapes for people to have a brain break. The hope is that these lead to improved morale and connections, especially for new employees who might not have met many people. Typically, these programs are initiated by someone within the Human Resources (HR) sector. Companies in the tech sector, or those with many young employees, are often interested in trivia or engaging how-to sessions, whereas corporate clients are looking for more robust informative sessions. I've found this too with government/UN-agency groups—they request in-depth research presentations because that is what feels familiar to their office culture, even though the whole reason for a new type of wellness session like this might be to change things up.

Standardizing measurements for employee well-being is hard in industries with a lot of staff turnover and not many resources put toward funding. This would be a great area for growth—experimenting with different types of workplace well-being programs and measuring impact over time.

Also, because virtual workshops are easy to schedule and share with staff, there is a growing need for more types of content. It has become a palatable office expense in many corporate cultures to set aside time for this type of engagement—and has become an "allowed break" in office scheduling to watch and/or participate in this type of thing. Providing value virtually is another good area of growth for people who want to participate in this space.

Meditation and mindfulness classes are readily available online these days, and easy to integrate within a workday without much disruption. A great study from 2019 showed that participants who did eight weeks of a guided body scan mindfulness practice showed decreased signs of biological and psychological stress compared to a control group. The benefit of these small but mindful habit changes is that they allow us to manage what is happening around us with less stress so that we can put our intentions and energies into work or causes or people who matter most to us. And we can prepare to try to plan for a dream workday. We all know that disruptions and changes happen regularly, and knowing how to stay mindful in those moments will help you navigate stress.

These are the new realities for employers struggling to stem the tide of employee burnout. Prioritizing mental health and well-being in the workplace offers a provocative framework for a revised business strategy anchored in compassion and support.

No one job policy can solve all our problems, but compassionate humans who manage other compassionate humans can examine the systems over which they have control and look for opportunities to make things better. If you are in a leadership or management position, I'd urge you to think about how decluttering can improve the quality of your staffs' lives, which can create a better functioning and organized work environment too. To do that, consider assessing how clutter effects the time and energy of your colleagues (and yourself!).

Informed by the results of assessments on workplace time and energy, here are some workplace decluttering ideas to consider implementing. Remember that if your position involves supervising others and encouraging office wellness, please consider implementing some of these ideas, for everyone's sake, including yours!

Some examples of ways to inspire workplace policies in support of decluttering are shared below. Add to these ideas based on your intimate knowledge of your work environment. Having a menu of options within these categories can help to identify which activities meet the needs identified during your assessments. Keep in mind that many of these options are cross-cutting in terms of the impact they can have on the lives of staff members.

- The exercises on time and energy should provide some data for your office to examine on when people feel most aligned with certain work tasks (emails, meetings, and such). Knowing this, consider having people share this information with others when scheduling tasks so theyare setting themselves up for success. As broader office policies, you may wish to start all meetings no earlier than 8:00 a.m. or declare one afternoon each week to be meeting-free.

Energy Assessment

Time Needed: 5–10 minutes per day for one week

Materials Needed: pencil/pen, paper

Prompt: How does your energy change through-out the day? Are there certain times when it feels best to work on certain tasks?

The purpose of this assessment is to figure out where your energy naturally peaks and dips throughout the day. Give yourself one week to pay careful attention to how you feel when doing your everyday tasks. You can write your notes in your calendar, your journal, or even the Notes app on your phone; any place is good as long as you can go back through to look for patterns of how your energy shifts throughout the day and by the type of task you are working on. The list of questions below can help prompt thinking about these activities in new ways. As always, write what comes to mind without censoring yourself.

Questions to consider:

• When are you most able to concentrate on one task at a time?

• When do you feel focused and alert?

• When do you feel sluggish?

• Are there times when interacting with people feels difficult? Easy? Engaging?

• How many hours of sleep did you get last night? Did the quality of your sleep impact your energy the next day?

After a week, or even longer if you can track for closer to a month, you may be amazed to see what patterns emerge.

Think about what you see coming through this assessment in terms of when you might feel most ready to declutter something or when you prefer to have time for rest and creative expression.

Continue reviewing your responses to assess what times are best for social connections, for regular sleep cycles, for creative projects, etc. If you can, hold yourself gently during the week of tracking and the follow-up search for patterns. There is no judgment needed: this is an aware-ness-raising exercise. We all have habits that we can adjust for the better. When our circadian rhythm, the natural energy arc for people throughout a twenty-four-hour period, isn't functioning well, we can become exhausted. Exhaustion can influence and compound mental health challenges, which puts people at higher risks of illnesses and disease.

After you've assessed your energy and time for at least one week—or, ideally, for thirty days—move on to the workplace version of this prompt and share insights with your team (if you work with others).

- Lenient staff leave policies can support people to not just attend health appointments, but also take the time needed to plan and schedule them. Health appointments can be inclusive of therapy, time to walk or exercise, or other ways the individuals in your workplace define their needs.

- If a health insurance and or Employee Assistance Plan (EAP) is part of your benefits package, look into expanding it to support the expenses of staff members by hiring professional organizers to help them or their relatives declutter. Many EAP plans offer support for child or elder care services, and this can be viewed as analogous to that type of activity. Particularly, as mentioned earlier in this book, with a rise in elderly hoarding rates more and more staff will need to have time and resources available to manage decluttering tasks for others.

- How does the physical workspace for your staff support their efforts? Incorporating wellness design in the office (group spaces or work from home situations) can add joy into the space, encouraging people to keep using it and interacting with the tools around them.

- David Allen noted that "all organizations should establish a purge day," where everyone has permission to spend the whole day in decluttering mode on their computer and in physical spaces, like offices or kitchens and break rooms, where you spend your time. Digital decluttering can also take place during these moments. Scheduling bulk clean-up days guards this time from competing priorities and can be scheduled based on consensus within your team—quarterly, monthly, or even weekly (typically weekly purge days are adjusted to be a few hours).

- Set up accountability hours where staff can come together (in person or virtually) and co-work on tasks of their choosing. They may elect to use this time for deep work (creative or intense work needing high concentration and minimal distractions) or for personal admin tasks which routinely clutter up to-do lists. This type of co-working is a form of "body doubling" where colleagues provide accountability and connection to one another while maintaining focus on their own goals.

Leadership Support for Aligning Energy and Work

Time Needed: 30 minutes, scheduled regularly

Materials Needed: pencil/pen, paper, virtual or in-person meeting space

Prompt: How can leadership teams support staff members and colleagues to manage clutter within the workplace by aligning work with natural energy patterns?

Being a leader within an organization is an opportunity to help everyone feel good about the work they are doing, at times that make sense, in spaces that are clear of clutter.

Set up a meeting with your leadership team to discuss how clutter affects time and energy within your workplace. You may wish to have an open discussion on the topics presented throughout this book. Ideally people will have had the chance to complete the Energy Assessment shared earlier in this chapter. This will give your team more data on how to consider people's energy and time as they relate to completion of work activities.

Consider questions like:

- What times are the best and worst to plan important meetings?

- Do certain people on your team need to protect their mornings so they can have deep work time when they are most focused?

- How much time do people need to do the tasks they are responsible for in the workplace?

- Can you allot one afternoon per week or per month for personal and communal decluttering and planning (virtual and tangible)?

- What are other ways you can support staff so they can align their energy and work to be in flow as much as possible?

Subsequent meetings with the leadership team can identify opportunities to address clutter in your workplace from different perspectives. At the end of your gatherings, collect your thoughts and decide the next best action steps to take toward becoming decluttered. Remember that when resources are finite, we must be careful to either declutter the number of things we are doing or the volume of any given task.

Feel free to adapt these exercises and reflection questions as needed if you work for yourself, do unpaid labor on behalf of yourself and your family in your home, or if any other descriptions of "leadership" and "workplace" resonate with you. How we view the workplace may be a personal definition, but digging into the clutter in these situations is universal.

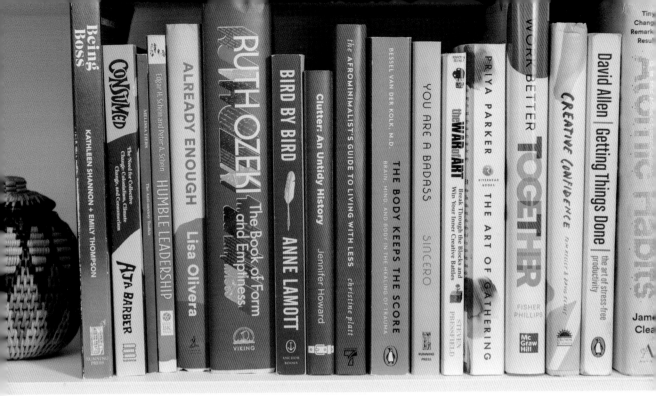

Clutter as a Metaphor

I hope that by now you're seeing clutter in ways beyond just the stuff you shoved in a drawer. Those feelings of being too busy or hiding what we want to say can be heavy and challenging to carry with us all the time. Many of these situations come up because of expectations from others or society that we internalize as sentiments we must manage alone. The longer we stay in a state of that inner congestion, the more our bodies get used to that feeling of being disconnected from what we really want in life.

Most health care jobs I had were like drinking from a fire hose. Each week there was a new emergency and new things to design or manage or respond to were added to your plate, usually without added staff to support the work or money to get things done. Public health as a discipline has an attitude of "let's solve this immense problem of poverty and global health crisis" with whatever meager resources we have been given. Yes, we would like more money and resources and political power, but darn it, we are going to try to change the world anyway without all of that. I felt personally responsible for the HIV epidemic in a country I wasn't from.

I was a short-term visitor, and I only had access to a certain amount of capital, financial and personal. Yet the mission-driven aspect of my work fueled me. It made me believe for a time that anything could be possible: why not try to see if things could be improved. But in reality, it was more than the system could handle—certainly more than I could handle.

The inflated sense of responsibility and mission may have had some elements of good in it—the value of wanting to be a helper in this world is one I agree with generally—but it also came from the egos and power trips of the institutions I worked within, something I was slow to understand during my twenties. In a race to achieve and cure and perform, the opportunity or urgency to pause and reflect is never treated as being of equal value as time. This disconnect manifests physically, emotionally, and environmentally for many of us.

When we devote too much time to work and community activities that are not the right alignment for us, we may feel fatigued. Conversely, when we find balance and engage in activities that align with our values, space, and time, we can experience joy, meaningful connections, and contentment.

In our earlier exercise on assessing our energy, we learned that we do certain tasks best at certain times of day. There are tasks that require intense focus, while others can be done with less rigor. Think about the tasks you do that require intense focus and concentration—make a list. And think of other things to do that may not be as rigorous—make a list of those also.

Most people can only focus in short bursts of time, so as you look at your calendar, protect the zones of the day during which you feel your most focused. Set yourself up for success by trying to do just one or two items from your list of tasks that require deep focus a day. As you practice this more, it may become easier to do longer blocks of focused time or more of them.

Often when we are overwhelmed with things to do, our anxiety spikes because we are mixing a variety of individual tasks (call this person, email that company, etc.) without clarity about what's important and when we are best placed to work on certain tasks. To declutter ideas (often cross-cutting through all areas of health, home, and beyond), we've got to work through a few things.

Through decluttering, which goals am I more able to meet?

Think back to the assessments you have done on your health, home, and beyond. Did you identify certain areas that needed more attention? Consider writing down your goals to align with those categories—for instance having an index card labeled: Health—Biomedical Goals. Under it you might have tasks like schedule telehealth session with primary care doctor, reach out to local yoga studio for intro student special, and so on.

When we see our ideas and tasks line up with goals we have based on needs we have identified, we are self-reinforcing that doing.

When will I schedule time to act on these goals?

Unless we do regular check-ins with our ideas, they get to live rent-free at the back of our minds forever, cluttering up space. Setting aside time to sit with them—make decisions, make forward progress—is key. Looking at your energy assessment of what you like to do when, consider using either some "open attention" time on your calendar to look at your ideas folder and either refine it to make things easier to find in the future, if you have decided to keep things, or let pieces go. You can take your favorite or most important ideas that need action and schedule them into your deep-work time blocks.

One exercise to try aligning your ideas to your goals is to take a stack of index cards and think through all the next best steps you have going on. For your "waiting to do" piles, label them with words that inspire action, such as *abundance* for money tasks or *vitality* for health. On the index cards write down the next steps you need to take to move toward that goal. Then when you pick the next thing to do from the pile, you can see how it aligns with your ultimate goal.

The more you practice decluttering what you have, the easier it becomes, because as you do it, you see how much of the important stuff you are keeping. But this requires a commitment to choose peace and ease over the volume of the stuff (ideas).

At the very least we want to examine our ideas, decide where they should live, choose how much volume in our lives they should take up, allocate time to deal with them, and then move forward.

Consider taking time each year to go through your papers (physical and digital) and other workplace ephemera and think about which projects or activities meant the most to you. A certain paper you wrote? An office policy you worked on? Making a collage or putting together an album (or a shadow box, vision board, etc.) with these items can be a great way to declutter. Look back at the earlier examples of creativity projects for more guidance on how to process these items.

Talking with a Boss

Time Needed: 15 minutes

Materials Needed: quiet space for a conversation between yourself and your boss

Prompt: Decluttering Work for Everyone

Often when I am working in a house where there is more than one adult, the responsibilities around decluttering and organizing are much lower for the adult whose job is deemed "too busy" or "too important." One approach to rightsizing this distribution might be a bottom-up approach, whereby responsibilities are divided using a tool like Eve Rodsky's *Fair Play*. Addressing things from a top-down approach—for the adult who feels they "cannot help"—traditionally would mean a discussion with a boss or manager figure to address this with whatever the blockage point is. These are some talking points in a script for a discussion that could take place, for instance, with the husbands who don't think they have enough time to spend helping their families create tools they can take to their employers, like scripts, so they can get the time they need—and if they are the bosses, they need to make those changes. I will say also, sometimes the person is their own boss, and they have to make a mindset shift that decluttering or reprioritizing time is intrinsically important enough that they will do it for their greater well-being. Although ultimately the right to manage your life and time should be valid and enough, many employers currently respond only to situations whereby the result is an increased element of productivity or output. While we work to change this dynamic in the long run, we may need to buy into that in the short term.

Here are some talking points:

- I'd like to bring up some issues around my availability to participate in my household responsibilities, which are affecting me in the workplace . . .

- I find my time and energy are cluttered at work because of . . .

- With more available time to deal with clutter at work I could . . .

- The lack of equity and participation is harming my relationships, which . . .

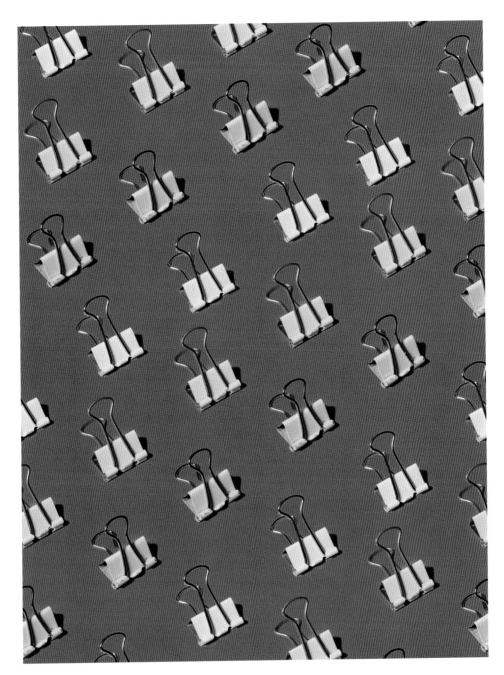

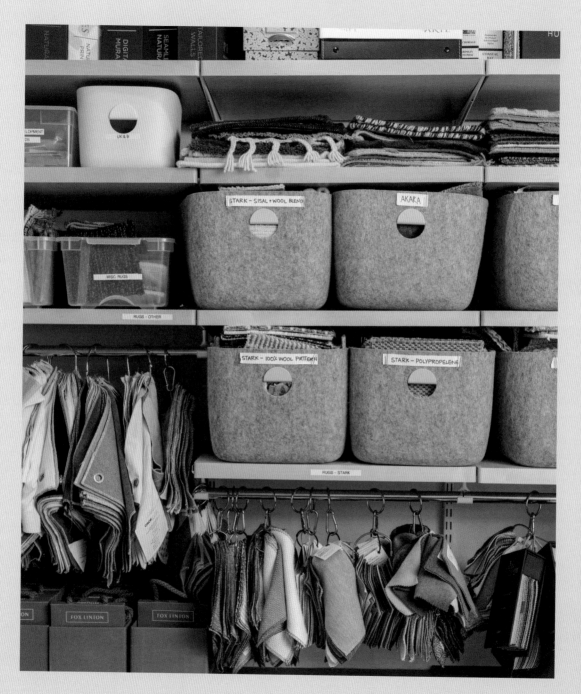

Case Study
Workspaces, Homes, and Beyond

In 2021, I worked at a design firm in Washington, DC, to organize their office space, a charming but narrow rowhouse in the design-centric Georgetown neighborhood. Their new office space was already bursting at the seams with samples, client project bins, and reams of paper were everywhere. Their design team needed a calm, inspiring workplace to access their creativity for their clients, but they found themselves distracted and overwhelmed by all the clutter. Designers shared insight with me along the lines of, "It's hard to envision beautiful spaces for my client when my own work environment feels messy." I can relate to this—as a professional organizer, when I go through waves of being extremely busy, and clutter accumulates in my mind or home, it makes it hard to declutter for my clients. Similarly, this firm needed support.

Clutter was leading to strained relationships between team members as they struggled to find the right samples and create beautiful spaces. Sustainability was also a core value for them, and we made a goal to reuse as many supplies as they had on hand and create a more functional system for using their office space to its fullest. But I knew from years of experience that a perfectly organized space is only helpful when there is a commitment from the people using it to maintain it. We needed a plan and an agreement.

To get the team started, I wrote an office-organizing manual for them with an overview of their systems and proposed habit changes; if people committed to the system and the behaviors, they might be able to thrive. Manuals and standard operating procedures are common in many traditional workplaces, and they are something that businesses (and even homes) I work with want to put in place because they help take the nebulous feelings of being overwhelmed. They also provide guardrails to parse out those concerns into categories and steps that feel manageable, especially when shared within a community.

My first goal in this manual is to understand and articulate the mission this ties heavily into our earlier discussions on mindful living and organizing. With the design team, we had a solid starting point because they already had a strong mission statement: "As a design firm, we consider all the work we do to be in pursuit of leaving the world a bit more beautiful than how we found it." With that in place, we could then connect the dots between their mission and their office environment. This manifested in their vision for an organized office: To create beautiful spaces for our clients, we must feel energized by our workplace too.

Creating and maintaining organized systems allows us to spend more time creatively designing and being efficient project managers and less time looking for things under piles (or other things that distract us from our goals). Because reducing our impact on the environment is a core value of our firm, we know that minimizing the surplus of materials we keep around (and taking good care of the ones we use regularly) allows us to keep our consumption habits low, which helps our planet.

With these principles in place, we could map out and list the categories of behaviors and habits and the types of stuff that would be encountered.

Standard Operating Procedures to Maintain a Beautiful and Organized Workplace

Staff Habits

- To support staff creativity but corral messy desks, everyone should be allowed to have one bin (or basket, tray, etc.) where they can keep special materials. This is the total amount of volume allowed on a desk though—if the container starts to overflow, items will need to be returned to the materials library or discarded.

- Before new samples are ordered, staff members should review the materials library to confirm that they are not already present in the office.

- Once client projects are completed, all materials should be returned to the materials library and/or discarded within one month.

Daily Tasks

- Staff will scan their desks and move any finished samples into the clear bins marked with category names (tiles, fabrics, wallpapers, etc.) in the materials library.

- Twice per week, the intern will take the clear category bins and rehome the samples in their designated bins/drawers in the materials library.

Weekly Tasks

- One-hour weekly desk reviews are a great way to maintain order in an office. This can be an agreed-on time when everyone does this together (for instance, Fridays at 3:00 p.m.) or a time in the week when everyone is expected to have spent an hour on their own doing this. (For instance, by 4:00 p.m. on Fridays, everyone should have completed this activity.) Weekly reviews can include putting away samples in their correct bins, filing paperwork, or other tasks as set by your office. It is important that this is time respected by managers and supervisors so that staff incorporate this into their regular work routines.

Monthly Tasks

- One afternoon per month a deep dive by category should be done whereby all the bins/drawers of any category (like fabric) are gone through to make sure the only samples kept are ones that are used and needed for your work. Samples should be folded or otherwise put back neatly at the end of this review. Over time these sessions will take less and less time because of the volume and importance of materials present. These reviews can be done passively during meetings (e.g., everyone sorts a bin of fabric during a staff meeting) or can be more of a "fun" office moment—music playing, teams trying to finish their reviews before other teams, and so on.

- The operations management team will schedule any pickups or drop-offs based on the output of the monthly review (e.g., drop off empty paint cans, have contractor remove broken/junk items, drop off items for client homes that are ready to go, etc.).

Quarterly Tasks

- One afternoon per quarter an office review of supplies, organization, and materials can be carried out to help maintain order in the environment. See above for examples of the monthly review but expand this beyond the categories living within the materials library.

Categories of Things to Organize

- **Fabric.** Fabric samples live in the white bins in the materials library. From left to right as you enter the room, bins should be sorted alphabetically by designer and then by color and pattern.

- **Wallpaper.** Wallpaper samples live in the magazine holders in the materials library. From left to right as you enter the room, holders should be sorted alphabetically by designer and then by color and pattern. The exception is the few holders at the start of the row, which contain multiple designer names.

- **Tile.** Tiles are currently stored in drawers on the left-hand wall system and in bins on the right-hand desk side. Ideally, they will mostly be stored in a center island to better account for their weight. They are sorted by designer or type (e.g., marble).

- **Wood.** Wood samples are currently stored in bins on the floor under the right-hand desk while they await being stored in a center island to account for their weight.

- **Paint.** Paint samples are in a bin on the floor because of their weight. Painted swatches of color are sorted by the two main companies used: Benjamin Moore and Farrow & Ball.

- **Carpet.** Carpet samples are stored in bins on the right-hand side of the room. They are sorted by designer and style.

- **Leather.** Leather (natural and vegan) takes up several drawers and bins on the left-hand side of the room.

- **Finishing touches.** Items like pulls, sample finishes, mirrors, and such are predominately stored in the top row of drawers on the left-hand side of the room.

Places to Keep Organized

- The materials library contains all samples that may be used to create client designs. Labels and order of materials may be adjusted once final storage bins arrive and staff have finished decluttering categories.

- The meeting room contains trays and drawers connected to client projects.

- The supply closet contains basic office supplies and consumables.

- The basement stores packages waiting to go to client homes, staging items, company documents, and heavy or irregularly used office products. Once cleared out it may contain a central island for storing incoming packages, a place to break down and store cardboard boxes, and excess trash (nonfood items).

While the above plan and standard operating procedure was particular for this design team, any type of office environment can commit to getting organized. Once you have a detailed plan and agreement in place, make sure there are clear communication strategies for new staff to onboard. It's also a good idea to set monthly action items and assign them to specific people (or teams) to implement the plan. That's why I recommend that staff in Human Resources or Leadership make sure to incorporate decluttering time into the weekly routine.

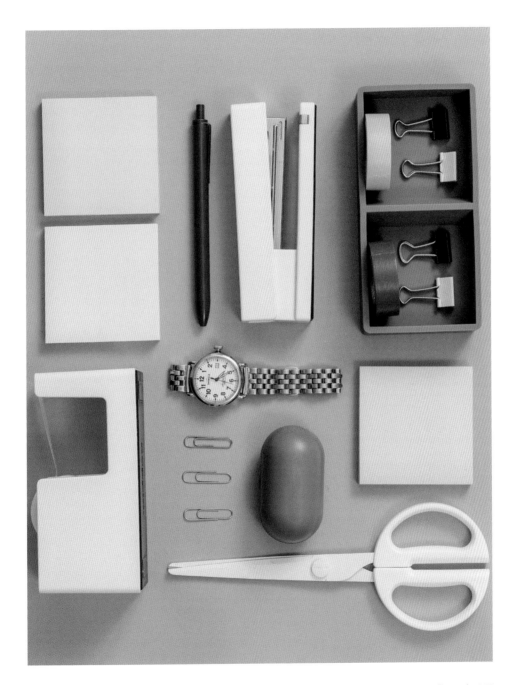

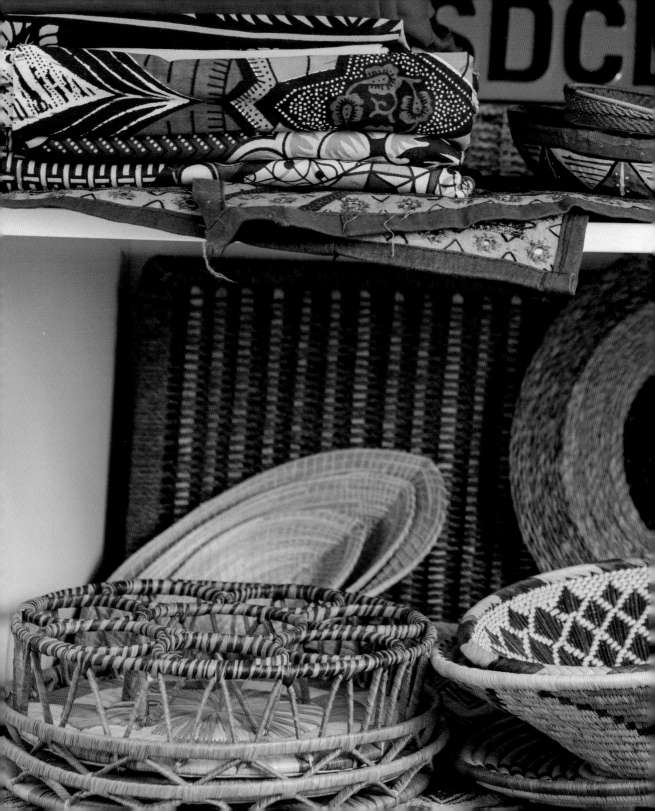

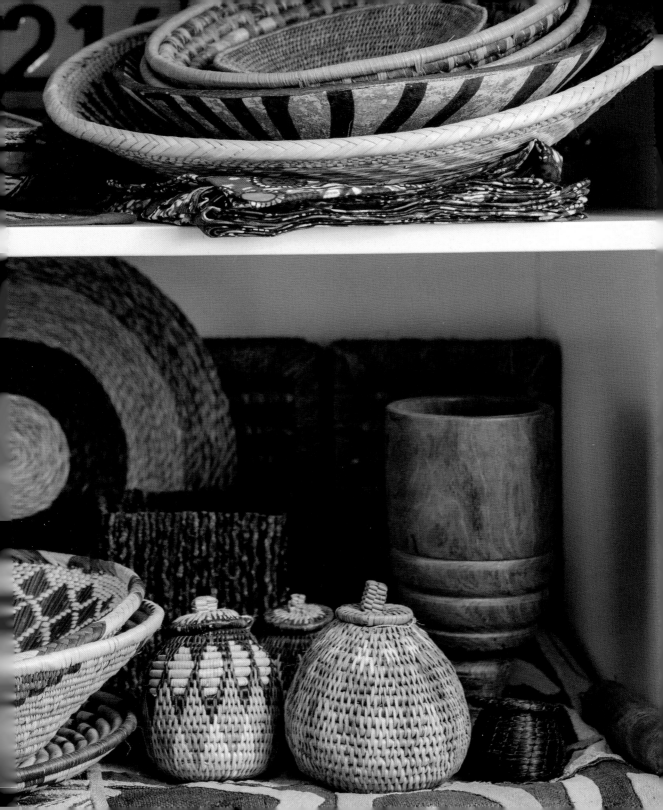

CONCLUSION

Mindful Organizing That Works

When I was six years old, my dollhouse figurines didn't get a lot of use; I was too busy rearranging the furniture and putting things away. Early signs of a professional home organizer, I guess—although I didn't have my first actual client until I was twenty-eight and living in Swaziland.

My first organizing job started with an offhand comment to a colleague at work: I could help you with that.

At a work meeting, we gathered around a wooden table, and Rachel, a senior manager at the US embassy, where I was working at the time—shared that the idea of packing up *all* her stuff was stressing her out. She knew that even with the state department's ten-thousand-pound packing allowance, she would be over her weight by the time the last box was sealed. "It's happened to me before," Rachel said, "with previous foreign service moves, and after three years in Swaziland, if anything, I've only accumulated more stuff." For Rachel, only having one more overseas post before she headed to DC to retire lingered in the back of her mind—and she dreamed of a much smaller home, unlike what she had been allowed and provided with in her various roles at the state department.

"I could help, you know, go through your things," I offered. Rachel raised her eyebrows at me and smiled. "Really?" I told her how I like that sort of stuff, and we quickly found a date to start. She suddenly seemed almost excited to get started. Almost.

In 2009 the idea of taking a few hours on the weekend to help my colleague made sense. What else would I be doing? In Swaziland during the week, I worked all day on HIV/AIDS programming. On Saturday nights, I drank lukewarm beers and on Sundays I did my nails and caught up on the week's papers. Rinse and repeat. A few afternoons with Sarah in her house would be a nice change, plus I liked moving things around and puttering through closets, trying to make sense of order and space before with my friends.

Rachel was a big boss at the embassy. Maybe twice my age at the time. I was just twenty-eight when I arrived and in the right place at the right time too. I became the youngest USAID country director anyone I met could remember. These days, the "30 under 30" list is the new "it" place to prove your competence, but in 2008, especially within USG ranks, youth was not revered. I was nervous to meet in the home of a seasoned foreign service agent heading toward retirement, let alone, communicating my ideas of what to do with *her* stuff. But I also was used to navigating the fear of a new challenge regularly.

My job scared me almost every day of the three years that I held it. The pressure was internally driven. (To quote Taylor Swift, "It's me, hi, I'm the problem, it's me.") This was largely because my commitment to mitigating the HIV/AIDS epidemic was personal. Ever since the loss of my uncle, who died from AIDS in 1993, all of my professional choices were personal. Isn't that how it works? We respond to life's curveballs and painful moments and try to do something about the chaos. Which is to say that right up until the day I went to meet Rachel to sort through her belongings, I was used to pressure. If anything, it was all I knew. An afternoon in an overflowing closet would feel like a vacation from my usual sort of pressure, right?

Having been at Rachel's house for one or two work events, I knew that there was a lot of stuff—it was a "full house," you might say. But at a party, you see what your host wants you to see: the piles and the stacks are tucked away into closets and behind closed doors. This day was different.

Rachel was anxious when I arrived, talking quickly, and gesturing wildly around the house. I assumed she was fixated on her upcoming move, but throughout the day, I realized it was more about the vulnerability she was experiencing by letting me into her home—deep into her home, not just the polished version of "dinner party presentation." Rachel's closets were packed with outfits she wanted to wear somewhere, someday, and figurines purchased in locations around the world. Each had a story to tell and sat in her home for years; unworn, untold, and gathering dust.

We spent hours sifting through her things, and eventually, some were packed away, and some were achingly let go. She hugged clothing that had lived on several continents with her one last time before dropping them into the donation bag. At one point, Rachel needed a break, and we sat outside drinking Coca-Cola and staring at the neat rows of hedges and spotting the occasional crow flying by. We were both exhausted. But deep within me, something else was awakening. I loved listening to Rachel's stories, hearing more about her life and how certain experiences shaped her beliefs around what she had held onto in her home. It was an early lesson on the way we collect memories and objects throughout our lives. I felt special gaining her trust and listening to this strong woman navigate objecthood, a life of traveling to various assigned locations, the absence of certain things, and the possibility of reimagining her relationship to clutter. I didn't intellectually know then how health, home, and work could all be related to clutter, but I was starting to feel it. For Rachel, it turned out that her relationship to clutter was deeply influenced by her relationship to work: the frequent moving made her want to gather reminders of all the places that, at one point, signified home to her. These reminders became her tools of comfort. Now that she was ready to retire into her dream home—a smaller home—she needed to reassess her relationship to all her stuff, not to mention the reassessment of work, purpose, and duty that would surface with retirement.

Spending that day with Rachel was a wake-up call for me. A warning sign of what could come if I surrounded myself with things and business to distract me from examining my true desires. *But what do I really want?* I wondered after combing through Rachel's home. I wanted less stuff, first and foremost. I wanted to be intentional with my home space and work environments. I also wanted to keep spending time with people to reassess and transform the cluttered areas of their lives.

For the next few years, while based in Swaziland, I turned to organizing the homes of my colleagues as one way to practice that intention. However, I ignored the inkling to follow that desire further than just a weekend hobby. For years, I continued waking up for a grueling work week, with days spent being told by others that I was failing at . . . everything. I kept drinking on Saturday nights, unsure of what else to do with my sliver of free time. I kept collecting items, hoping they would mean something one day. And yes, eventually, I woke up to my intuitive, healing self, who knew something needed to change. This self knew I needed to start decluttering my life.

For many of us getting decluttered is transformational. As empowering as change can be, it can simultaneously raise concern. When you stop a habit that has led to clutter, like purchasing too much or allowing too many unused items to be in your home, you may feel a sense of withdrawal. This can be very painful because your body has become habituated to buying things or feelings of being stressed out all the time, and this can often present itself as resistance to change. Other people feel lighter in their surroundings and with their daily tasks. Keep an eye out for any biological symptoms you experience while decluttering—not with judgment, just an eye toward awareness. Change can feel hard. It creates discomfort in our bodies and minds. Resilience is an important strength to cultivate to adapt to the realities of the times. Resistance to change passes with time and repetition. With all these changes to facets of your life, it's important to monitor how you feel along the way and adjust as needed.

As we turn to the final pages, let's all take a deep breath and turn inward for a moment. Life can be overwhelming. Navigating through long work schedules or balancing work, home, and maybe even homeschooling, it's easy to fall into the trap of convenience and chaos.

Take the time to understand and address the bidirectional impact clutter has on your health, home, and other areas of your life now—before you are in a state of being overwhelmed, you will increase your well-being measurements. You don't have to do it if you don't want to, but you'll want to have done it before long. Just one next best step at a time.

I hope this book has helped you on how to identify—and then act on—priorities in your professional goals, your work environments, and even within yourselves so that you feel better prepared to balance your life and live with intention every day. When considering your life and a desire to mindfully organize and declutter that which doesn't serve you, you may want to try different ways of thinking through problems and solutions. That's what happened with the clients I shared about during this book.

- For Sara, by mindfully organizing her paperwork she felt more in control of her physical and financial life;

- For Beth, decluttering in her home led to more open discussions with her mother so they could work through their shared loss together;

- And for Peter, by letting go of some of the ideas that had been stealing his focus he was able to be more present when his first child arrived.

And for me?

When my boyfriend broke up with me a few months after I started my professional organizing business, he emphasized that we hadn't been sparking joy for each other. (I had just started my KonMari career, so at least he was on brand.) It was hard to hear, even though I knew he was right. For a time, we had been happy enough to live beneath some piles of unspoken truths and to sidestep our real wants. We settled for a "good enough" relationship. The thing about decluttering though—the hard, figuring-out-what's-going-on-inside-me type of decluttering—is that once you get started, you no longer feel like allowing possessions, or even relationships, that don't work for you to exist in your life anymore.

Two years and fifty-one weeks after that breakup, my now-husband, Jason, proposed with a list of things that spark joy for him. If I agreed, my marrying him would be number one. He didn't know the wording of my previous breakup, but for me it was so poignant. Marie had been right: saying good-bye to things that don't spark joy creates space for those that do. Now, decluttering doesn't always lead to romantic love, but it helped me reassess all the parts of my life and, yes, find my person.

Decluttering is not about getting rid of everything in your life. Taking things that are not helpful to you out of your life adds more to your well-being. Thousands of hours in people's homes have shown me how public health starts with the stuff around us and within us. I went around the world and wound up in my neighbors' closet to examine how and where we live and work affects our personal sense of power and well-being. As I said earlier, I needed to learn these things in a new way—to be able to feel and experience them so that I could integrate and change internally, not just on an intellectual level. Mindful organization helped me rewire my experience with the world so that I could be better positioned to enjoy my health, my home, and beyond—and I hope it does the same for you.

ACKNOWLEDGMENTS

Thank you to the clients I've worked with, those I sat with in clinics, and those I decluttered with in closets. Your stories informed who I have become and the messages in this book.

Thank you to Sarah Warner and Dan Crissman, who thought I could do this even before I did. I am grateful to you and the teams at Indiana University Press and Red Lightning Press for the opportunity to create and publish this book.

Thank you to the Zoe Feldman Design firm for allowing photography of your office space to appear in this book. Thank you as well to my client SP for supporting the photography in her home.

Thank you to the friends, colleagues, and family members who have cheered me on from country to country and from one professional path to another.

Birch Thomas, your creativity and compassion inspire me. Thank you for bringing my ideas to life so beautifully through your photography.

Allie Rigby, when my sentences were piles of mismatched words and phrases, you helped me find the underlying messages I had hidden beneath them. Thank you for decluttering my chapters and mindfully guiding me on this writing journey.

Jason Hughes, your love overwhelms me in the best possible way. Thanks to you, and Huck, for creating a space where I felt supported enough to grow toward my dreams and write this book. You are my heart, home, and beyond.

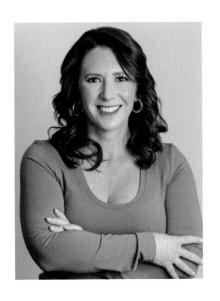

JENNY ALBERTINI has been organizing health systems and closets around the world for more than two decades. At thirty-six, she left a high-flying career in international health to train under Marie Kondo and became one of the first certified KonMari consultants, and she focused on finding joy within piles of clutter. While putting in thousands of hours of professional organizing, Jenny has been featured on PBS, on NBC, in the *Washington Post,* on Apartment Therapy, and in many other media outlets. Recognized for her work fighting the AIDS epidemic while waging war on clutter, she has found a unique way to infuse public health into the professional organizing field. Now, nearly a decade into her career transition, Jenny's first book guides readers through how decluttering mindfully can improve our well-being. She lives in Washington, DC.

For Indiana University Press

Lesley Bolton, Project Manager/Editor

Tony Brewer, Artist and Book Designer

Dan Crissman, Editorial Director and Acquisitions Editor

Samantha Heffner, Marketing and Publicity Manager

Brenna Hosman, Production Coordinator

Katie Huggins, Production Manager

Dan Pyle, Online Publishing Manager

Jennifer L. Witzke, Senior Artist and Book Designer